Psychiatric Aftercare

PSYCHIATRIC AFTERCARE

PLANNING FOR A
COMMUNITY MENTAL HEALTH SERVICE

MAX SILVERSTEIN

Philadelphia
University of Pennsylvania Press

PREFACE

About 325,000 persons are admitted as patients annually to public mental hospitals in the United States. Less than half are first admissions; 175,000 are readmissions.

Each year about 310,000 patients leave the public mental hospitals. They undertake the hazards of living again, as ex-patients, in the community. More than half will return, at some time, to hospital. The highest proportion will return within the first year after release. Mental health workers, planners, and administrators hold that many more ex-patients would sustain community tenure if appropriate follow-up aftercare services were available to them. But no one is sure to what extent this is so.

This book is a report of a study of certain aspects of the aftercare problems of over 10,000 patients released from public mental hospitals. It highlights major aftercare service needs of released patients, the availability of aftercare services, the utilization of these services by ex-patients, and the relationship between utilization of services and community tenure.

While the study was conducted in Pennsylvania, its findings may have significance for planning and program development in other localities. Every state and major community in the United States is currently engaged in implementing comprehensive community mental health plans. The planning process was initiated by the action of the United States Congress in 1963 when funds were appropriated to the states for this purpose. In 1965, Congress allocated the first installment of money to construct comprehensive, community mental health centers.

The community mental health center is at the heart of the bold new approach to mental health programming. It is

v

conceived as the all-purpose complex of related services designed to meet the full spectrum of mental health need, from diagnosis and treatment to rehabilitation and aftercare. In 1967, about 285 centers will be operating in the United States, serving a population of approximately 50 million people. By 1970, 580 centers are envisioned. The Congress has committed itself to appropriations of significant sums to accomplish these ends, not only to help in the construction of community facilities, but also to assist in paying for professional and other personnel to man the centers. From 1965 to 1970, the sum of $335 million has been assigned for construction of community mental health centers across the nation with a further $140 million for personnel costs. Additional millions of dollars, from state and local sources, will help underwrite the cost of community mental health center programs throughout the nation. By 1975, 2,000 centers are planned to serve the total population.

A study which can throw light on the nature and extent of patient aftercare requirements in a community mental health program should be an important tool for workers, planners, and administrators. It is hoped that this study to some degree fulfills this need.

In sum, the study provides answers to the following questions:

1. What are the specific aftercare needs of released patients?
2. To what extent are aftercare services available?
3. To what degree do ex-patients utilize aftercare services?
4. Does utilization affect community tenure?

These questions, in researchable form, and tentative answers articulated as hypotheses will be found on pages 127-129. The results of the study raise additional questions about long-held notions and assumptions concerning the problems of aftercare for discharged mental hospital patients. New hypotheses are formulated for further testing.

The book is divided into two parts: Part I reports major statewide findings and interpretations. Part II focuses on background, methodology, and data specifically applicable to planning regions and service areas within the state. Readers interested primarily in the broad overview of aftercare may find Part I useful in itself. For those interested, in addition, in the planning process, technique of assessment, comparative data, and analysis, Part II may be a helpful supplement.

From 1952 to 1966 I served as executive director of the Pennsylvania Mental Health Association Inc., a statewide voluntary organization of lay and professional persons concerned with policies and programs having to do with mental health services. From 1962 to 1965, I was actively associated with the Pennsylvania official mental health planning process, with a special assignment in the study of aftercare. In addition, I served as chairman of the Governor's Committee on Employment of the Mentally Handicapped, as well as consultant to the Task Force on Aftercare of the State Comprehensive Mental Health Planning Project. From these vantage points I was able to help design and carry through efforts to identify the aftercare problem firsthand, and to gain an understanding of it.

I am indebted to many professional persons who helped along the way, especially to John Davis, Joseph Adelstein, William Camp, Sylvia Green, and William Miller, of the Office of Mental Health, Pennsylvania Department of Public Welfare; to Lucille Pflaumer, research associate, Office of Research and Planning, Pennsylvania Department of Public Welfare; and, to the members of the Task Force on Aftercare; James Harris, Martin Adler, Homer Capparell, John Goldschmidt, Roy Hackman, David Landy, Saul Leshner, John Phillips, Maurice Reisman, Irvin Rutman, and Alfred Wood, Jr.

Finally, I wish to express my gratitude to Julius Jahn, Director of the Research Center, University of Pennsyl-

Preface

vania School of Social Work, who guided me through the design and analysis of this research.

July, 1967   MAX SILVERSTEIN
University of Pennsylvania
School of Social Work
Philadelphia, Pennsylvania

Contents

PART
I

The Nature of Psychiatric Aftercare

CHAPTER
1

INTRODUCTION

Aftercare has become a discrete term in the mental health glossary. It is viewed as a process of providing services to assist the mental patient *in the community* after his inpatient psychiatric treatment(1).

Aftercare achieved high-priority attention in the United States beginning in 1955. This was the year of the dramatic reversal of the upward trend in the number of patients resident in mental hospitals. The discovery and widespread use of the psychopharmaceutical drugs, the increase of personnel-to-patient ratios in hospitals, the increased provision of alternative community services, including outpatient clinics, day care centers, psychiatric units in general hospitals—all contributed to this phenomenon(2).

However, one disquieting trend began to appear and has continued during the past twelve years. While the discharge rate was going up, the *readmission* rate also was climbing. Prior to 1955, most admissions to mental hospitals were first admissions. By 1963, only 47% of all admissions were first admissions(3). Zubin's analogy is apt: the mental hospital can be likened to a subway train, ". . .

3

always filled but never the same people, although the same passengers get in and out at various time periods"(4).

It was natural that heightened attention was directed toward the problem of aftercare and its relationship to community tenure of ex-patients. The reports of the United States Joint Commission on Mental Illness and Health(5) and other studies stressed the development of community-based psychiatric services, including the aftercare program for the discharged patient in the community. The bold new approach to mental health programs envisioned in the Commission's final report, and urged upon the Congress by the late President Kennedy in 1963, is contained in that appealing phrase "the comprehensive community mental health center." The center's principal motif is provision of "continuity of care" through easy access to and transfer between facilities best able to meet the changing treatment needs of the patient. Equally cogent is the shift in emphasis from institutional to community care which the center epitomizes.

PURPOSE OF THIS STUDY

The primary purpose of this study was to analyze the aftercare needs of patients leaving the eighteen state mental hospitals in Pennsylvania, in order to provide a planning basis for meeting those needs in the Pennsylvania Comprehensive Community Mental Health Plan(6).

A major objective of the Comprehensive Plan is the development of integrated community-based mental health services, of which aftercare is one ingredient. Eight planning and service regions(6) were established within the state, to serve as the locus for the major facilities to be developed under the plan. (See Chapter 7 for description of regions.)

The results of this study provide specific data on which regional aftercare programs can be based. It makes available specific knowledge of the number of patients who

4

will be returning in a given time period from state hospitals to each region, what their specific aftercare needs will be, to what extent services now available in each region can meet these needs, and what modifications and additions in the present aftercare program of each region are required.

SOURCES OF DATA

Two primary sources of data for the study were used for analysis: the "Task Force Report on Aftercare" of the Comprehensive Plan, and the "Aftercare Study of Patients of State Mental Hospitals," conducted by the Office of the Commissioner of Mental Health, Department of Public Welfare, Commonwealth of Pennsylvania, at the request and under the general direction of the Governor's Committee on Employment of the Mentally Handicapped.

The Task Force Report is essentially a position paper on the subject of aftercare, representing the collective professional opinion of ten selected authorities and practitioners in psychiatry, psychology, sociology, social work, vocational rehabilitation, and social agency administration. The report represents the professional dimensions of an aftercare program. It proceeds on a number of assumptions drawn from previous studies and a literature search, develops a statement of principles and program recommendations, and in general serves as the theoretical base and conceptual model for the development of the aftercare phase of the Comprehensive Mental Health Plan.

The Aftercare Study was designed to identify selected characteristics of every patient leaving the eighteen state mental hospitals in Pennsylvania in one year (see Appendix: *Schedule*). It included recordings made by hospital staff on the aftercare services needed and recommended for each patient; the community facilities required to provide the services, both those available and those not available; the work potential of each patient, and related data. It also included a follow-up recording of all study patients who returned to hospital within a one-year period after leaving (see Appendix: *Schedule*).

The study period began on October 1, 1962, and ended September 30, 1964. The study patients were defined as those who left the hospital from October 1, 1962, to September 30, 1963. All study patients who returned within a 12-months period after date of discharge were included in the "returns" data and analysis.

Primary responsibility for recording data on the schedules rested with the director of social work at each hospital. The overall study itself was managed and directed by the State Office of Mental Health.

Definitions of Aftercare Services

The selection and definition of specific aftercare services used in this study were derived from two sources. First is the working definition(7) developed by the Task Force report of the Comprehensive Mental Health Plan. Second is the description of specific aftercare services developed by the Aftercare Study as a result of the pretest, one-month trial study.

The Task Force defines three broad program categories of aftercare services: (1) medical services, (2) social services, and (3) vocational services.

Medical services include all phases of medical supervision, medication management, periodic medical review, and emergency service.

Social services are those services aimed at restoration of social skills, with special reference to enhancing the process of community reintegration. Among these services are: (1) casework and group work services, supportive counseling, assistance with living arrangements, income maintenance and other health and welfare services; (2) specialized resocialization services, both residential and non-residential.

6

Vocational services include all efforts to reestablish the patient as a self-supporting economic unit. Among these services are vocational diagnosis, evaluation and guidance, sheltered employment, reeducation and special education services, job counseling, job finding, and job placement services.

The pretest trial study, conducted over a period of one month, involved seventeen state hospitals. The directors of social service of each of the hospitals, in cooperation with the other "discharge staff members," recorded data on a schedule. A preliminary analysis of returns was followed by a series of conferences with the directors of social service. Out of this experience, a selection was made of the ten most frequent aftercare service recommendations. Other items were added to the schedule and these became the forms used in the final one-year study.

For purposes of the Aftercare Study, the following specific aftercare services, based upon the pretest trial study, were selected to be included for analysis: regulation of medication, psychotherapy, counseling, sheltered living arrangements, resocialization, vocational rehabilitation, day treatment center services, public health nursing, Public Assistance, and Alcoholics Anonymous (see Appendix: *Schedule* for definitions).

DATA COLLECTION

The study design, research instruments, procedures of data collection, and techniques of analysis are generally consistent with other follow-up studies of mental patients.

Most aftercare studies to date have observed the study population in the posthospital milieu. The observers or judges generally were extramural, community-based personnel. The population in this study is observed, measured, and classified at the critical point of discharge by hospital staff. The same observers and judges made the observations and classifications at the point of return—a second critical point in the total mental health care sequence.

The design is meritorious in certain respects, but also has its defects. It is assumed, for example, that the treatment team of the hospital—the psychiatrist, psychologist, social worker, nurse, rehabilitation counselor—has a reliable collective judgment on the aftercare needs of the patient, based on its working knowledge over a relatively long period of time. It is further assumed that the hospital staff, particularly the social service and rehabilitation staff, has working knowledge of aftercare resources in the communities to which the patients return, as well as knowledge about the familial and living arrangements in which the patient will take his place after leaving the hospital. Similar assumptions are made with regard to the method of observation and the selected observers when the patients return to the hospital. A staff decision on readmission of a patient must be reached; knowledge of the precipitating conditions and reasons for readmission are necessary in making this decision. These data were recorded on all study patients who returned to hospital. In short, the validity of the data rests on the value placed on the judgments of hospital staffs.

The reader is no doubt aware that clinical judgments with respect to mental illnesses generally do not yet meet the highest tests of precision. The findings, therefore, have intrinsic limitations. The importance of hospital staffs' judgments, on the other hand, should not be minimized. For the patient, these judgments are crucial.

The primary instruments used were the Appendix schedules referred to above. Instruction sheets for completing the schedules, definitions of terms, and refinements in the schedules themselves were developed as a result of the pretest. Consultation with hospital superintendents and other staff was held to define the purpose of the study and the methods to be used in the statistical reporting procedure. Each hospital designated one staff person to record the data and act as consultant on any possible questions.

A coding system was developed, making it possible to transfer data to IBM cards. For purposes of this study, selected data on study patients are tabulated.

AREAS NOT COVERED BY THIS STUDY

It is recognized that the answers to the research study questions still fall short of providing an analysis of the total problem of aftercare.

One limitation is obvious. While the study design includes data on study patients who returned to the hospital, there is no provision for data on those who do not return during the one-year period following release. A comparative analysis of these two groups would obviously yield significant information. This gap was recognized and a research proposal was developed early in the study period to undertake such a study. For a variety of reasons, this was not done, but there is evidence now that it will be undertaken under the auspices of the Office of Mental Health.

In addition, there are a number of broad considerations with which this study does not deal. First, it should be pointed out that the "staying-out" index, expressed as the percentage of total discharges who have remained in the community for a certain length of time, is crude, misleading, and could be misused. If misused, it could tend to place a premium on keeping people out of the hospital and strengthen the belief that rehospitalization is a failure to be avoided at all costs. From the point of view of the patients' welfare, rehospitalization may be actually thought of as part of an effective aftercare program at a particular point in time. This conventional measure of success—the capacity of a program to prevent patients' return—therefore has limitations.

Second, in dealing with utilization of aftercare services, the related problems of effectiveness and costs are

9

important—and they are not covered in this study. It does analyze the actual utilization problem as revealed by data on "returned" study patients. In so doing, the study may bring into sharper focus the nature of this problem.

Related to utilization is also the question of patient motivation. Mental health literature refers continually to the difficulties of bridging the gap, not only between the hospital and community services, but also between the ex-patient and the community's aftercare program. The Task Force Report cites the problem of lack of motivation on the part of ex-patients, indicating that special devices must be built into aftercare programming to take this factor into account. Labeling the condition does not, of course, provide an answer. The analysis of the data of this study opens up possibilities for raising significant additional questions on utilization; further research might answer these questions.

Third, while this study deals with aftercare needs and aftercare services, it does not focus on the vital connections required between these services. It is clear that a major concern in aftercare programming is continuity of service and coordination of aftercare services. The problem of coordination in community care is not unique to mental health. Yet related studies reveal that the situation in psychiatric aftercare is especially acute, since a large proportion of discharged patients require more than a single type of service. The data obtained from this study throw additional light on this aspect of aftercare.

Finally, this study does not attempt to approach the overall critical problem of public attitudes toward the mentally ill. These attitudes can play an important part in developing the climate and context for a community-based aftercare program. This matter is treated with considerable intensity in the report of the Joint Commission on Mental Illness and Health. The "rejection cycle," as it is referred to in the report, must be taken into account in any community aftercare plans and programs. This is especially true since,

10

according to the Joint Commission report and evidence re-vealed in other studies (8), community health and welfare agencies, as well as professional and learned groups directly related to mental illness, tend to join the general public in rejecting the seriously mentally ill and particularly the pa-tients in state mental hospitals.

REFERENCES

1. Southern Regional Education Board and National Institute of Mental Health. *Aftercare: Report of a Conference on an Assessment of Needs and Problems in Aftercare,* Paul W. Penningroth and Dorothy Sparer, Eds. (Atlanta, Ga.) October 1963.

2. Felix, Robert H. "Breakthrough in Mental Illness," *Health, Education and Welfare Indicators* November 1963, pp. XXXV and XXXVI.

3. National Institute of Mental Health. "Patients in Mental Institutions, 1962, Part II. State and County Mental Hospitals," (Washington: U.S. Government Printing Office) 1964, pp. II-8 and II-9.

4. Freeman, Howard E. and Simmons, Ozzie G. *The Mental Patient Comes Home.* (New York: John Wiley and Sons) 1963, p. 44.

5. Joint Commission on Mental Illness and Health. *Action for Mental Health.* (New York: Basic Books) 1961.

6. Commonwealth of Pennsylvania. "The Comprehensive Mental Health Plan." Clifford J. Bodarky, Ed. (Health and Welfare Building, Harrisburg, Pa.) 1965.

7. Commonwealth of Pennsylvania, Office of Mental Health, Department of Public Welfare. Position paper: "Rehabilitation and Aftercare for Mentally Ill and Emotionally Disturbed Adults," (Harrisburg, Pa.) October 1964.

8. Jacob, Norma P. "Why Do Community Psychiatric Clinics Reject Patients?" Unpublished paper presented at annual meeting, American Orthopsychiatric Association, New York, N.Y., March 19, 1965.

CHAPTER
2

The Patients Who Leave

Nine out of ten patients who left the eighteen state mental hospitals in Pennsylvania during the study period required one or more specific aftercare services, in the judgment of the hospital staff.

During this period there were 10,786 releases; 633, or approximately 6%, of the study patients were released from the hospital more than once during the study period. Of the total releases, 1,137, or 10.5%, were judged not to require any aftercare services.

For the remainder, there was a total of 16,824 recommendations for specific aftercare services, indicating, among other things, that a substantial number of patients required more than one type of aftercare service. Table 1 shows the frequency distribution of aftercare service recommendations for study patients.

Living arrangements and employability status of study patients at the time of release help fill out the profile of "patients who leave." As shown in Table 2, the majority of released patients, approximately 75%, will reside with kin; of these, over one-third will live with spouse, and a little over 40% will live with other relatives.

13

TABLE 1
NUMBER OF TIMES SELECTED AFTERCARE
SERVICE RECOMMENDED FOR STUDY PATIENTS

Aftercare Services	Number of Recommendations	Percentage
TOTAL	16,824	100.0%
Regulation of medication	7,574	45.0
Counseling services	3,180	18.9
Psychotherapy	2,192	13.0
Vocational rehabilitation	1,048	6.2
Alcoholics Anonymous	688	4.9
Public Assistance	636	3.8
Resocialization services	614	3.6
Sheltered living	441	2.6
Public Health Nursing	83	.5
Day treatment services	48	.2
Other	320	1.3

Data on job readiness and employability status of study patients at the time of release, as shown in Table 3, indicate that less than half, 5,190, or 47.3% of the study

TABLE 2
STUDY PATIENTS' LIVING ARRANGEMENTS
AFTER LEAVING HOSPITAL

Living Arrangement	Number of Releases	Percentage
TOTAL	10,786	100.0%
With relatives	4,384	40.6
With spouse	3,847	35.6
Live alone	826	7.6
Transferred to other institutions	632	5.8
With nonrelatives or foster family	568	5.2
Other	148	1.3
No report	181	1.6

patients will enter the labor market and presumably seek employment.

About 30% of the patients who will be entering the labor market will be returning to jobs held prior to hospitalization. Approximately 64% will be seeking new positions.

Hospital staff judgments on the job readiness of the released study patients who will be entering the labor market (Table 3) indicate that 39% are considered good employment risks and a little over half (52.7%) are considered fair employment risks. Five percent are considered poor employment risks.

Of the total 10,786 releases during the study period, 5,678, or 52.7%, will not be entering the labor market. Distribution of reasons for patients not entering the labor market is shown in Table 4.

TABLE 3

STUDY PATIENTS WHO WILL BE ENTERING THE LABOR MARKET,
JOB READINESS, EMPLOYABILITY STATUS AT TIME OF RELEASE

	Number	Percentage
TOTAL	5,190	100.0%
Returning to former position:		
Yes	1,525	29.3
No	3,299	63.7
No report	366	7.0
Job readiness:		
Poor	258	5.0
Fair	2,662	52.3
Good	2,068	39.0
No report	202	3.7

CHARACTERISTICS OF AFTERCARE NEEDS

The findings reveal certain significant characteristics of the aftercare needs of patients who leave.

1. With respect to medication, it was to be expected

15

TABLE 4
REASONS FOR STUDY PATIENTS NOT
ENTERING LABOR MARKET

Reasons	Number	Percentage
TOTAL	5,678	100.0%
Household duties	2,185	38.5
Physical or mental disability	1,422	25.0
Age	879	15.5
Institutionalized after leaving hospital	494	8.7
Inability to adjust to employment	220	3.9
No report	478	8.4

that a substantial majority of patients released from mental hospitals would be placed on a continuing prescription of psychotropic drugs. The Task Force Report estimated that 60% of the patients would be placed on psychotropic drugs at release(1). The unofficial consensus is that from 80% to 90% are released with continuing drug prescriptions.

The results of this study indicate that the proportion lies between the 60% estimate and the unofficial 80–90% figure. For the total 10,786 releases, 7,574 "regulation of medication" recommendations were made. This is 70.2%.

2. Three aftercare services—medication, counseling, and psychotherapy—constitute over 75% of the aftercare recommendations for study patients. In these three categories there were 12,946 recommendations out of the total of 16,824. These are not only the most frequently recommended but also indicate that, in the judgment of hospital staff, three out of four patients who leave require continuous medical-social treatment. In short, the notion that patients who are released are "well" or "recovered," in the sense that those who have had a hospitalization for a physical illness are "well" and may require only some convales-

cent care, can easily be abandoned. For three out of four patients who leave the hospital, it can be said that their treatment is being continued, with only their status changed from inpatients to outpatients.

3. The findings raise a perplexing question with respect to social and vocational services. Briefly, how does one account for the relatively low frequency of recommendations in the area of vocational rehabilitation, resocialization, and related services? The assumption has been that the released patient, while his needs for medication and psychiatric supervision would be substantial, would require, equally, social and vocational services to help his reintegration into community living. Forrest *et al.* conclude, as a result of a study of 3,000 mental patients over a ten-year period, that over 50% of even severely ill, chronic mental patients can be *socially* rehabilitated through drug therapy(2). Medication is assumed to serve to alleviate symptoms so that social and related services could become operative. The data suggest that hospital staffs do not think along these lines when releasing patients.

4. An unexpected finding is the very low number (6%) of released patients who are referred for public assistance services. Given the relatively high rate of unemployability of released patients and the assumed low level of income, it could have been expected that a much higher frequency for this recommendation would result. Miller and Dawson(3) in the California study of 1,045 released patients residing in the community, found that 85% of these patients came from the *lowest* socioeconomic class, with 27% dependent upon public assistance. Since in Pennsylvania the mental health program and the public assistance program are both operated by the same Department of Public Welfare, lack of communication or "red tape" cannot be considered as contributing to this result. This may indicate that the overwhelming majority of patients who leave state hospitals are above the indigent socioeco-

nomic category. If the patients who leave are representative of all state mental hospital patients, then it could further be concluded that patients in state hospitals are, for the most part, not indigent. This, of course, would run counter to the findings of studies on social class and mental illness(4).

One can speculate, on the other hand, that patients with available economic resources are more likely to be released; those who are indigent are more likely to remain in hospital. A follow-up study on this point might yield some interesting results as to what proportion of patients stay in state hospitals for economic rather than psychiatric reasons.

5. The finding that three out of four released patients will live in the community with spouse or relatives is significant. It would seem to cloud part of the image that families "forget" or "abandon" the mentally ill member. On the other hand, however, it might indicate that it is precisely those patients whose families do forget or abandon them who remain in hospital. A comparative analysis of those who leave hospital and those who stay, on this question, might be worth pursuing.

6. The fact that only 5% of released patients live in foster families or with nonrelatives indicates that low priority attention has been given to this method of providing suitable living arrangements for patients who could profit from them. Experience in other states, notably Maryland and California, shows that a significant number of patients could be released from hospital to appropriate foster family homes. In Maryland, for example, approximately 1,500 hospital patients annually are placed with foster families on release, as compared to the 220 Pennsylvania patients of this study.

7. Although over 10,000 patients are released annually from Pennsylvania state hospitals, less than half are candidates for employment, and, of these, almost 30% will be returning to their former positions. This leaves a total of

about 3,300 released patients who may require assistance in finding appropriate employment and keeping it. The fact that only approximately 1,000 released patients were referred to vocational services (see Table 1) would indicate that hospital staffs feel that 2,300 can fend for themselves in the marketplace for jobs. There may be some question that this is actually so. It would be of interest to examine this particular aspect of the reemployment problem further. This examination could proceed on the assumption that

TABLE 5

AVAILABILITY OF AFTERCARE SERVICES
RECOMMENDED FOR STUDY PATIENTS

Aftercare Services	Total	Available	Not Available	Percent Not Available
TOTALS	16,824	16,287	537	3.1
Regulation of medication	7,574	7,565	9	0.1
Counseling services	3,180	3,013	167	5.2
Psychotherapy	2,192	2,036	156	7.1
Vocational rehabilitation	1,048	1,036	12	1.1
Alcoholics Anonymous	688	671	17	2.4
Public Assistance	636	636	0	—
Resocialization services	614	490	124	2.0
Sheltered living arrangements	441	421	20	4.5
Public Health Nursing	83	83	0	—
Day treatment services	48	16	32	66.6
Other	320	NR*	NR*	—

*No Report

vocational counseling, guidance, rehabilitation, and job placement services could be extended profitably to three times the number of released patients presently being referred for these services.

CHARACTERISTICS OF AFTERCARE SERVICES

Services to meet approximately 97% of all aftercare recommendations were judged by the hospital staff to be available for study patients, statewide.

As shown in Table 5, there were 537 instances reported in which aftercare services were not available to fulfill 16,824 recommendations. Only in the day treatment center category was there a significant deficit reported in which the lack of available services exceeded in number the services available.

On a statewide basis, the principal providers of available recommended aftercare services for study patients are the state mental hospitals themselves. The hospitals are expected to provide, through medical, psychiatric, and social work professional staff, almost one-half (48.7%) of the recommended aftercare services. Table 6 shows the facilities to which study patients were referred for recommended aftercare services and the number of recommendations made to each facility.

It is clear that, in substantial measure, the aftercare program for released patients is a function of the state hospitals. Only in a limited way can there be said to be a community-based aftercare program in the Commonwealth. If the major thrust of comprehensive mental health planning is to provide community facilities close to home, then, for all practical purposes, to achieve this goal, the program is starting almost from scratch.

Part of the ideology of community-based facilities with respect to aftercare has to do with strengthening the released patients' connections with "normal" modes of living—that is to say, with separation from the hospital

20

TABLE 6
WHO WILL PROVIDE RECOMMENDED AFTERCARE
SERVICES TO STUDY PATIENTS?

Resource	Number	Percent
TOTAL	16,287	100.0%
State hospital	7,938	48.7
Private physician	3,869	23.8
Bureau of Vocational Rehab.	971	6.1
Alcoholics Anonymous	668	4.0
Public Assistance	636	3.9
Ex-patients' club	259	1.6
Community clinic	249	1.5
Social agency	207	1.3
Church	126	0.8
Nursing home	107	0.6
Family care	104	0.6
VNA or Public Health Nurse	83	0.5
County home	60	0.3
Community center	46	0.3
Clergy	34	0.2
Halfway house	25	0.1
Day treatment center	16	—
Other	291	1.7
No report	130	0.7

milieu. If, as the findings reveal, released patients in great numbers continue in aftercare under the auspices of the hospital, the goal of separation is delayed and may be more difficult to achieve.

On the other hand, there may be cogent and practical reasons for state hospitals to accept the responsibility for providing aftercare services to released patients. One important consideration here is that hospital staffs who have treated patients in hospital have a familiarity, knowledge, and grasp of the patients' needs and, therefore, would be perhaps in better position to help meet them. This connection may also have value for released patients. They have

21

"experienced" the hospital staff which helped them through a critical period of their illness. In short, separating aftercare services from hospital services may result in severing a helpful relationship between staff and patient which, in the last analysis, is the key to effective treatment.

Both these considerations—the value of separation and the value of continuity—should be weighed in planning comprehensive aftercare services for released patients.

It is important to note, however, that community psychiatric clinics throughout the state, on the whole, do not provide services for patients released from state hospitals. There are 104 full-time and part-time community psychiatric clinics in Pennsylvania. These are primarily voluntary organizations, financed by private funds. However, sixtyfour of these clinics receive state financial assistance in the form of grants to help meet operating costs. The latter stateaided community clinics receive, on the average, 50% of their operating budgets from state funds. It is altogether reasonable to expect that these clinics would undertake, in some substantial way, to provide continuing psychiatric treatment and supervision to residents of their own communities who have returned from state hospitals. It is, therefore, striking that only 1.5% of study patients were served by community psychiatric clinics out of the total 12,946 recommendations for medication, counseling, and psychotherapy.

Finally, the fact that the findings of this study reveal such a high level of availability raises an interesting question. To what degree do hospital staffs recommend aftercare services for released patients on the basis of existing facilities? Contrariwise, to what degree are aftercare services not recommended, although needed by released patients, because hospital staffs know that such facilities do not exist? In planning the study and preparing hospital staffs for completion of schedules, the point was underscored that recordings should reflect hospital staff judgments as to patients' needs, irrespective of availability of resources to meet them. There appeared to be every assurance that this directive would be followed. There still remains a lingering doubt, however, since both the findings on aftercare needs and availability of aftercare services appear to be so far removed from expectations.

REFERENCES

1. Commonwealth of Pennsylvania. "The Comprehensive Mental Health Plan." Clifford J. Bodarky, Ed. (Health and Welfare Building, Harrisburg, Pa.) 1965, p. 69.

2. Forrest, F. M., Geiter, L. W., Steinbach, M. "Drug Maintenance Problems of Rehabilitated Mental Patients," *The American Journal of Psychiatry*. July 1964, Vol. 121-1, p. 33.

3. Miller, Dorothy, M. A. "Worlds That Fail: Part I. Retrospective Analysis of Mental Patients' Careers: Part II. Disbanded Worlds: A Study of Returns to the Mental Hospital," *California Mental Health Research Monograph,* No. 6 and No. 7 (State of California, Department of Mental Hygiene, Bureau of Research) 1965, p. 45.

4. Hollingshead, A. B. and Redlich, F. C. *Social Class and Mental Illness.* (New York: John Wiley & Sons) 1959.

CHAPTER
3

THE PATIENTS WHO RETURN

This chapter deals with three related questions. First, the proportion of patients who return to hospital within one year after release; second, factors which primarily precipitated patients' return; and, third, aftercare services which might have prevented patients' return.

Before proceeding with a discussion of these questions, it may be useful to review the method used to collect data on study patients who return to hospital. Each patient who left the eighteen state mental hospitals, from October 1, 1962, to September 30, 1963, was included as a study patient. During this period, the data on each study patient was recorded at the time of release (see Appendix: *Schedules*). If a study patient was readmitted to hospital within a 12-month period after date of his release, selected relevant data were recorded on the return study schedule (see Appendix: *Schedules*). The study period for returned patients ended on September 30, 1964, so as to give each released patient a full 12-month period of observation. In short, the full study time extended over a 24-month period.

THE RETURN RATE: PRECIPITATING FACTORS, PATIENT EXPERIENCE

From October 1, 1962, to October 1, 1963, there were 10,786 releases from the 18 state mental hospitals. A total of 8,005 did not return during a period of 12 months following release; 2,781 returned during the 12 months following release. The statewide rate of return, as expressed by the percentage of releases, was 25.7%.

For each study patient who returned within 12 months from release date, hospital staff recorded, following the readmission conference, the major reasons for patients' return. For the 2,781 returns, 3,012 factors were cited which, in the judgment of hospital staff, primarily precipitated patients' return.

Table 1 shows the frequency distribution of the return

TABLE 1

FACTORS WHICH PRIMARILY
PRECIPITATED PATIENTS' RETURNS

Factors	Number	Percentage
TOTAL	3,012	100.0%
Inability to cope with stressful situations	1,055	35.0
Refused or discontinued medication	414	13.7
Negative family environment	283	9.4
Excessive drinking	208	6.9
Premature release	197	6.5
Other environmental problems	183	6.1
Recurrence of previous symptoms	169	5.6
Different symptoms from previous illness	80	2.7
Other	172	5.7
No report	251	8.3

factors. Over one-third (35%) cited "inability to cope with stressful situations," a relatively nonspecific factor.

What effect would the provision of aftercare services for study patients have had on the return rate? This retrospective question was included in the schedule for returns and, for each returned patient, hospital staffs made a judgment and recording.

TABLE 2

AFTERCARE SERVICES WHICH COULD HAVE PREVENTED
PATIENTS' RETURN TO HOSPITAL

Aftercare Services	Number	Percentage
TOTAL	2,080	100.0%
Regulation of medication	589	28.3
Counseling	301	14.5
Psychotherapy	273	13.1
Day treatment center	224	10.8
Alcoholics Anonymous	155	7.4
Sheltered living arrangements	154	7.4
Vocational rehabilitation	118	5.7
Resocialization services	114	5.5
Other	118	5.7
No report	34	—

For 1,550 returns, the hospital staff judged that the provision of aftercare services would not have affected the outcome. In other words, for over half of the returned patients (55.7%), their rehospitalization could not have been prevented by the provision of aftercare services, in the judgment of the hospital staff.

For the remaining 1,231 returns, hospital staffs judged that the provision and utilization of 2,080 aftercare services by patients could have prevented rehospitalization. The frequency distribution of these services is shown in Table 2.

Approximately 60% of the total fall into the combined categories of medication, counseling, and psychotherapy. Vocational rehabilitation and resocialization services are at the low end of the frequency scale, together representing 11% of the total.

An unexpected finding is in the day treatment services category. In the data on patients released, only 0.2% of the total recommended aftercare services were for this service. For returned patients, the hospital staff judged that 10.8% of the total aftercare needs of returned patients, while out of hospital, were in this category.

The employability status of returned patients while out of hospital corresponds in most particulars to the employability status of the total study patient group. It will be recalled that about one-half of the 10,786 releases—5,190, or 47.3%—were expected to enter the labor market and presumably seek employment. For the returned patients, the proportion is 49.5%—1,376 out of the total of 2,781 returns—who were judged to be employable while out of the hospital.

TABLE 3

REASONS RETURNED PATIENTS DID NOT ENTER LABOR MARKET

Reasons	Number	Percentage	Percent of Total Study Patients (5,678)
TOTAL	1,405	100.0%	100.0%
Household duties	469	33.4	38.5
Physical or mental disability	531	37.8	25.0
Age	174	12.4	15.5
Institutionalized after leaving hospital	21	1.5	8.7
Inability to adjust to employment	56	4.0	3.9
No report	125	8.9	8.4

28

The important consideration here, of course, is the efforts made by returned patients to obtain employment while out of the hospital. This aspect of the problem will be discussed in the next chapter, in which an attempt is made to analyze generally the utilization of services and facilities by released patients who return.

For the 1,405 returns who were judged to be out of the labor market—that is, not employable, in this context —the frequency distribution of the reasons is shown in Table 3.

There are a few items in Table 3 which should be noted. Returned patients who were unemployable for physical and mental reasons constituted 37.8% of the total, as compared to 25% of all study patients. This is perhaps to be expected since the fact of their return would confirm that a higher proportion would be registered in this category.

An interesting finding is that only 1.5% of returned patients were institutionalized while out of the hospital. This item includes nursing homes, county homes, and jails. The fact that so few discharged mental patients found themselves in serious trouble with the law would suggest that some of the popular notions about ex-patients being a "danger to society" may be unfounded in actual fact.

A number of questions are raised by the findings on returned patients:

1. One out of four patients released from Pennsylvania's state mental hospitals is readmitted within one year. The statewide return rate is 25.7%, as compared to the national return rate of between 35% and 38%. What are the possible interpretations that can be placed on the relatively low return rate?

The most heartening interpretation could be that the Pennsylvania hospitals, comparatively, are performing at a higher rate of excellence in the treatment program for patients, so that those who are released are better equipped to sustain community tenure. While this would be a welcome deduction, a number of related facts make it necessary to question it. The findings of this study itself indicate that three-fourths of the patients who leave the state hospitals require continued psychiatric and medical supervision. While this factor in itself is not controlling, it is indicative. More telling are the facts about the state hospitals, described in Appendix: IV, indicating severe shortages in treatment personnel and considerable overcrowding.

In this connection, it might be well to cite the findings of California(1) and Massachusetts(2) aftercare studies. The California study revealed a return rate of approximately 40%; the Massachusetts study, approximately 33%. While there are no absolutes in comparing the quality of treatment between hospitals, there are a number of indices which throw light on this subject. In the California hospitals, there are 1.6 physicians per 100 resident patients; in Massachusetts, the figure is 1.27. In Pennsylvania, the comparable figure is 0.62.

In California, the professional patient-care personnel per 100 resident patients is 6.6; in Massachusetts, it is 7.9. In Pennsylvania, it is 5.6.

In California, the number of full-time employees per 100 patients is 38.3; in Massachusetts, it is 45.0. In Pennsylvania, the comparable figure is 35.4.

In California, the average daily maintenance expenditure per resident patient is $7.17; in Massachusetts, it is $6.80. In Pennsylvania, the comparable figure is $5.50.(3)

Using the above indices as criteria for judging quality of program, it would be difficult to attribute the lower return rate in Pennsylvania to excellence of hospital treatment. California and Massachusetts, with relatively higher return rates, appear to be equipped to provide a higher quality of inpatient treatment.

A second interpretation of the Pennsylvania return

rate could be a gloomy one, in reverse of the above—namely, that conditions in the Pennsylvania hospitals are so poor that patients and their families resist seeking readmission, even when indicated. (It should be added in this connection that many studies, including the California and Massachusetts studies, attribute to the families of released patients the crucial role in the decisions about readmission).

A third possibility is that the so-called "open door" or "revolving door" policy which seems to characterize the operation of many state mental hospitals throughout the country has not been as operative in Pennsylvania. The main thrust of this policy is to make it as easy as possible for patients who are released to return for periodic hospitalization as part of their recovery and treatment plan. It could very well be that in Pennsylvania, with the chronic shortage of staff and the overcrowding in the majority of its hospitals, hospital staff attitudes about readmission may be more rigid than would otherwise be the case.

A fourth possibility is of a different kind. This has to do with the degree of tolerance of deviant behavior in the community where the released patient is attempting to sustain tenure. There is no evidence, of course, to support the notion that the degree of this tolerance is either higher or lower in Pennsylvania, as compared to the rest of the country. It is mentioned here as a possibility because it is to this variable that many related studies attach great significance in the assessment of reasons for readmissions. Since the Pennsylvania return rate is considerably below the national rate, research into the meaning of this finding might be worth pursuing, perhaps using the above assumptions as a point of departure.

Finally, it is necessary to repeat what was alluded to in Chapter 1—that the "staying-out" index, as any kind of measure of effectiveness, has serious limitations and any importance ascribed to it should be done with caution. This is particularly so in light of the California study's finding that, while approximately 40% of released patients return within one year, the return rate is 70% in a five-year span.

2. One of the most important findings has to do with the relatively high frequency of need for day treatment center services of those study patients who return, as compared to the total released patients. It will be recalled that, in the judgment of hospital staffs, released patients had practically no need for day treatment center services after leaving the hospital. On the other hand, in assessing the aftercare services which may have prevented rehospitalization, this service is recorded at 10.8% of the total, involving 224 returned patients.

Once again, the data show, with respect to aftercare needs of returned patients while out of hospitals, that vocational rehabilitation and resocialization services are at the lowest end of the frequency scale. This confirms the results of judgments made on all released patients.

On the other end of the scale, there is confirmation that regulation of medication, counseling, and psychotherapy—comprising approximately 60% of aftercare needs of returned patients—are, as with all released patients, the predominant aftercare service needs.

3. The findings indicate that 13.7% refused or discontinued medication while out of hospital. This is a considerably lower rate than might have been expected. A number of studies(4) subscribe to the idea that the majority of patients who return "break down" because they discontinue their medicine. The chairman of the "Drug Committee" of the Pennsylvania State Office of Mental Health, a hospital superintendent, says in a private communication:

> . . . returns . . . would be reduced substantially if the patients would continue the medication as ordered by the doctor.

Leaving the matter of "how many" to one side, there are conflicting views on why patients discontinue or refuse

32

the prescribed drugs. One view is that the expense is prohibitive for many patients. A recent study(5) on this subject calculates that the average monthly retail medications cost to released patients is $18. Fifty percent of the returned patients in the county studied were living in families with income of less than $4,000 per year. The study concludes that these patients "would find it extremely difficult, if not impossible, to purchase the required medication."

The contrary view, again quoting the Drug Committee chairman, is:

> . . . patients stop medication for totally different reasons, the most prominent of which are either that they feel so well they do not think they need more, or the direct opposite, that they are beginning to relapse and refuse medication when offered by the family. Especially in the first case, the patient and the family tend to rationalize and say that they cannot afford to get the prescription refilled, when in fact they could very easily get the medication free if they were motivated to request it . . .

Perhaps the most vital consideration growing out of the findings reported in this chapter is that, in the judgment of hospital staffs, over 40% of patients who returned might have retained community tenure if they had received appropriate aftercare services. If these judgments are valid and the suggested recommendations had been carried through, the return rate would have been reduced by that proportion. Such an outcome would obviously have great significance.

The question arises, in light of the high degree of availability of aftercare services reported in Chapter 2—a rate of 97%—what prevented the provision of these aftercare services to returned patients? This leads to a consideration of *utilization* of aftercare services by returned patients, treated in the next chapter.

REFERENCES

1. Miller, Dorothy, M. A. "Worlds That Fail: Part I. Retrospective Analysis of Mental Patients' Careers: Part II. Disbanded Worlds: A Study of Returns to the Mental Hospital," *California Mental Health Research Monograph,* No. 6 and No. 7. (State of California, Department of Mental Hygiene, Bureau of Research) 1956.

2. Freeman, Howard E. and Simmons, Ozzie, G. *The Mental Patient Comes Home.* (New York: John Wiley and Sons) 1963, p. 44.

3. These comparative data are taken from the 1964 edition, "Fifteen Indices," Joint Information Service, American Psychiatric Association, and National Association for Mental Health, Inc., Washington, D.C.

4. National Institute of Mental Health, U.S. Department of Health, Education, and Welfare, Public Health Service. "Research Activities," (Bethesda, Md.) December 1964. p. 7.

5. Mental Health Association of Erie County, Aftercare Committee. "A Program to Provide Psychotropic Medications to the Impoverished Mentally Ill," (Erie, Pa.) October 1965.

CHAPTER
4

This chapter addresses itself to two questions: First, what is the utilization of available aftercare services by returned patients while out of hospital? Second, what is the relationship between patient utilization of available aftercare services and readmission of released patients? To deal with the latter question, comparative data from planning regions are used. (Regions are described in Chapter 7.)

It has been established that there were 2,781 readmissions during the study period and that, in the judgment of hospital staff, the utilization by 1,231 returned patients of 2,080 aftercare services could have prevented their rehospitalization. For 1,550 rehospitalized patients (55.7%), utilization of aftercare services would not have affected their return, in the judgment of hospital staff.

What are the principal reasons aftercare services were not utilized by 1,231 returned patients? Some important clues to the answer to this question are indicated in Table 1.

It should be kept in mind that the data refer to the problem of utilization of aftercare services by *returned pa-*

TABLE 1

REASONS AFTERCARE SERVICES WERE NOT UTILIZED
BY RETURNED PATIENTS WHILE OUT OF HOSPITAL

Reason	Number	Percentage
TOTAL	2,080	100.0%
Patient refused service	904	43.4
Service not available	419	20.1
Service not provided soon enough, or provided irregularly	326	15.7
Ineffectual planning	191	9.2
Other	112	5.4
No report	128	6.1

tients only. They cannot be used to characterize, therefore, the utilization problem of all study patients. They can, however, indicate the nature and extent of the problem as it occurs for a vulnerable proportion of all patients who leave hospital.

It will be noted at once that for this group of study patients the "availability rate" is 79.9%, as compared to the availability rate of all study patients of 97%. More significant, of course, is the finding that 43.4% of the reasons for nonutilization of aftercare services is the "patient refused service" category.

It is also worthy of note that there appears to be equal "failure" on the part of patients and the agencies expected to meet their needs, to account for lack of utilization. Of returned patients, 43.4% refused to be served; and 45% of the reasons for nonutilization were either for nonavailability of services or noneffectiveness of service operations.

A more precise picture, for purposes of this part of the study of the utilization of *available* aftercare services, requires that the "service not available" category be deducted from the total. The result is that, statewide, the net number of available aftercare service not utilized by returned patients while out of hospital is 1,661.

THE RELATIONSHIP OF UTILIZATION AND RETURNS

A true test, of course, of the retrospective judgment of hospital staff on the question of whether the utilization of available aftercare services would, indeed, have affected the return rate, would be an analysis of the experience of a comparable sample of study patients who did *not* return to hospital. Since these data are not available for this study, a second-choice test will be made, employing the comparison of return rates of regions and the rate of nonutilization of aftercare services of returned patients in each region.

Before proceeding with this test, it may be well to cite data available (Table 2) on return patients' attempts to obtain employment while out of hospital. It will be recalled that, of the total returns of 2,781, 1,376 were judged to be employable while out of hospital. These data on efforts to obtain employment by return patients while out of hospital may add a dimension to the question of the relationship between utilization and returns.

As can be seen in Table 2, over one-third (36.1%) employable returned patients did not seek employment while out of hospital. The lowest proportion in this category was in Region VI, which registered at 20.9%; the highest in Region III, with 58.0%. It can be assumed that not seeking employment and refusal to use available aftercare facilities are in the same or related order of behavior.

Now to return to the question of relationship between utilization and return rates. To analyze this relationship, it was necessary to assign a rank order of the computed return rate for each region. It was also necessary to compute a nonutilization rate for each region and to assign each region a rank order.

The rank order of regional return rates, from the highest to the lowest, is shown in Table 3. The rank order of regional nonutilization rates, using the "corrected figure," is shown in Table 4. The relationship between the rates of return and nonutilization is shown in Table 5.

TABLE 2
RETURNED PATIENTS' ATTEMPTS TO OBTAIN
EMPLOYMENT WHILE OUT OF HOSPITAL, BY REGIONS

| | Statewide | | | | | Regions | | | |
		I	II	III	IV	V	VI	VII	VIII
Total employable	1,376	236	95	57	53	48	105	654	118
Number who did not seek employment	497	81	29	33	20	19	22	252	31
Percent who did not seek employment	36.1	34.3	30.5	58.0	37.7	39.6	20.9	38.5	26.3

The initial formulation of the hypothesis stated that the higher the utilization of available aftercare services, the lower the rate of return to hospital. The hypothesis to be tested, restated, is that the higher the rank order of the nonutilization rate, the higher will be the rank order of the return rate. The tables were set up, for comparison pur-

TABLE 3
RANK ORDER OF RETURN RATES, BY REGIONS

Region	Return Rate (%)	Rank Order
VIII	27.9	8
VII	27.3	7
III	26.7	6
II	26.1	5
VI	24.5	4
V	24.4	3
I	24.0	2
IV	19.5	1

poses, in rank order from highest to lowest—i.e., the region with the highest return rate was assigned rank 8, and the region with the highest nonutilization rate was assigned rank 8. The hypothesis will hold if, as the rank order in

TABLE 4
NONUTILIZATION RATES BY REGIONS

Region	Total Returns	Did Not Utilize Available Aftercare Services	Non-utilization Rate (%)	Rank Order
V	143	120	83.9	8
VIII	224	169	75.4	7
VII	1,198	816	68.1	6
III	186	122	65.6	5
I	445	241	54.1	4
VI	190	78	41.0	3
II	237	70	29.5	2
IV	156	45	29.4	1

TABLE 5

RELATIONSHIP BETWEEN NONUTILIZATION
RATES AND RETURN RATES

Region	Nonutilization Rates; Rank Order	Return Rates; Rank Order	Outcome of Test
V	8	3	—
VIII	7	8	+
VII	6	7	+
III	5	6	+
I	4	2	—
VI	3	4	—
II	2	5	+
IV	1	1	+

nonutilization rate rises, the rank order of return rate also rises. As can be seen, in Table 5, there were five instances (marked "+" in "outcome of test" column) out of the eight in which this was the case.

It is clear that a relationship does exist between non-utilization of available aftercare services and return to hospital; that patients who leave hospital are more likely to sustain "community tenure" if they make use of available aftercare services.

Complete data, of course, are not available on all study patients with respect to their utilization of aftercare services while out of hospital. The data are based on hospital staff judgments about study patients who *returned* to hospital. The findings on utilization refer to approximately one out of four of the study population. It cannot be assumed that the returned patients are "representative" of total study patients. What can be assumed is that this group of study patients deserves high-priority attention in planning and programming aftercare services.

With the above provisos in mind, the following generalizations are suggested by the findings:

1. Utilization of available aftercare services by study

patients while out of hospital represents a major problem in that 44.3% of returned patients did not utilize aftercare services. One-fifth of these services were not available. This means that over one-third (35.5%) of study patients who returned did not utilize *available* aftercare services.

2. It has been established that, on the basis of this study, there is a relationship between nonutilization of available aftercare services and returns. It is recognized that the results are not overwhelmingly conclusive; they are generally consistent, however, with the proposition that aftercare services can, if used, help released patients sustain community tenure.

3. The study has indicated a number of problems requiring further research. The first is the matter of patients who refuse service. There has been extensive speculation on this phenomenon. All studies of posthospital patients' careers report it; and, as a matter of fact, in the literature it has been given a name—"the failure syndrome"(1). More often the phenomenon is described as "low-level motivation." There is no doubt that in order to make any aftercare program effective, better methods must be found to help patients make use of what is available.

These data reveal two important findings in the area of "low-level of motivation" on the part of the released patient. First is the finding that, statewide, 43.4% of returned patients who did not use aftercare services refused service. When this is coupled with the second finding that 36.1% of employable returned patients did not seek employment while out of the hospital, the problem assumes widespread proportions. Any plans for the development of effective aftercare services, whether based primarily in the state hospitals, in regions, in local communities, or in a combination, must have a built-in system for overcoming the gap between availability and utilization.

A second problem highlighted is the fact that 25% of the reasons that available aftercare services were not utilized

41

by returned patients had to do with the failures of the agencies and facilities involved in the referral to and provision of aftercare services. Again, this is a theme which is repeated consistently in studies of aftercare.

4. The high incidence of breakdown in the aftercare system goes to the heart of the question of coordination of resources in the interest of the patient. More important, without correction of the systemic defects, the goal of a continuum of care cannot be achieved. It is quite easy for even the most adept and practiced users of community health and welfare services to find themselves falling in between the slats, so to speak, of professional and agency programs. For the ex-patient this presents rough waters. The released mental patient, dropped into this turbulence from the relative predictability, integrated and outerdirected life of a state mental hospital, may find it extremely difficult to navigate. He may, in this struggle, seek the refuge of the "failure syndrome" as a more manageable and satisfactory solution.

Again, it is necessary to emphasize that any plan of aftercare, in addition to a built-in helping process focused on utilization, must provide for close links and easy access between its parts.

A study of the aftercare system in Allegheny County(2) confirms that it is "somewhat unstructured," with a lack of "feedback" between its components. This study also adds another dimension—the person in the system—through intensive interviews and follow-up of 34 released patients (out of the study population of 113 ex-patients). A few excerpts from these interviews may throw additional light on the "failure syndrome."

The ex-patients speak:

> "I'm lonely. No one to talk to—no place to go."
> "I hate hanging around, killing time—it's killing me."
> "If I don't get a job soon, get some routine in my life, I'll probably be back in."

"I'm turning night into day and day into night and it doesn't matter."

"You get up early; there's everything to be done and done and done and done—if you have anything to do."

"I feel close to my aunt, but I don't know if she feels close to me . . . I need someone to feel close to me, too."

Here are seven released patients telling of their loneliness, their sense of purposelessness, their need for human connection, and their thinly veiled nostalgia for the hospital. The hospital was a human society in which they were a vital part. It was in hospital that *people*—staff and other patients—had some functional and purposeful place in the patient's daily scheme of things, the patient in theirs. Fromm-Reichmann's "On Loneliness"(3) is perhaps the most definitive and illuminating description of "real loneliness" which leads ultimately to the development of emotional paralysis and psychotic states. *Ex-patients may, in fact, be seeking to sustain their health in edging back to a more accepting human society—the hospital.*

5. Finally, the findings on returned patients' attempts to obtain employment while out of the hospital give rise to a number of considerations. Obviously, if over a third of the employable group did not seek employment, it would be important to know much more than these data reveal about the nature of this circumstance. Levinson(4) calls work the "psychological glue" which holds a man together.

Was the failure to seek employment related to other breakdowns in the patient's posthospital world? It is conceivable that not seeking employment could only be one symptom of a recurrence of illness or other disablement. It is also quite possible to speculate that fear and anxiety made it difficult for the patient to seek employment, and that his very reluctance and failure brought forward other symptoms which led to the need for rehospitalization.

Since work is considered to be such an essential part of the employable ex-patient's rehabilitation, providing, among other things, self-esteem and a connection with his society, it would be important to undertake further research to discover the precise nature and extent of the reemployment problems faced by employable patients who leave state hospitals.

6. In any discussion of the released patient and his work, we come full circle to the central problem of public attitudes about mental illness and the mentally ill. Mention has been made previously about the level of toleration of deviance—or, put in another way, the ability of "significant others" in the patient's life to live with and accept "difference." In the larger circle of "significant others" we find the employer and the co-workers. What is their level of tolerance and acceptance of difference? Given the social stigma that is attached to mental illness, it is understandable that many released patients would not want to risk the potential rejection, isolation, and rebuffs that seeking and holding employment might entail.

Many ex-patients, in trying to reconnect with the work world, have found it expedient to deny the fact of their illness. What this denial, or "passing," costs the released patient in terms of self-esteem and integrity is hard to measure, but no doubt it is high.

As a result of a study of the attitudes of 200 employers in the Greater Boston area toward ex-patients and a subsequent study of patients leaving three state hospitals, Olshansky discovered the widespread planned practice of patient denial of illness. Olshansky reports(5) that:

> The majority of patients leaving mental hospitals recognize the fact of stigma and attempt to deal with it by passing—i.e., by keeping secret the history of mental hospitalization in their day-to-day transactions outside their immediate families . . . whether professional personnel like it or not, this is the road followed by most released mental patients. . . .
>
> Passing may involve some anxiety for those who practice it, but this anxiety is probably considerably less

44

than that produced by identifying oneself as an ex-mental patient and testing out and suffering the many kinds of response that persons of varying sophistication and sensitivity offer.

This, then, could be what life is like to a released patient: a lonely, tough and continuing contest with the sometimes unyielding and unwelcoming world of the "well." Admission to this world, also, may require lying about hospitalization. Could the hospital world be not only more secure but also a more honest world? The "failure syndrome" begins to make sense. An aftercare program or system of services, however plentiful and varied, which does not deal effectively and creatively with the individual in the system —this person who is fighting to become a member of the "well" world, with all its faults—has missed the main chance.

For the main chance in aftercare is the creation of maximum possibilities for the released patient to become a vital part of the human society of his choice. By so doing, the ex-patient not only can utilize fully the resources of that society, but also can help shape its character.

REFERENCES

1. Margolin, R. J. "The Mental Patient Who *Wants* to Fail." *Rehabilitation Record.* December 1962. (Vocational Rehabilitation Administration, Washington, D.C.)

2. Strecker, Mary C. and Dean, Charles W. "A Study of Patterns of Service to Persons Following Psychiatric Hospitalization in Allegheny County, Pennsylvania," United Mental Health Services of Allegheny County, Inc., April 1964.

3. Selected Papers of Freida Fromm-Reichmann. *Psychoanalysis and Psychotherapy.* Dexter M. Bullard, Ed. (Chicago: University of Chicago Press) 1959.

4. Levinson, H. "What Work Means To A Man," *Think.* January-February 1964, p. 7.

5. Olshansky, S. "Passing: Road to Normalization for Ex Mental Patients," *Mental Hygiene.* January 1966, Vol. 50, No. 1, (National Association for Mental Health, Inc., New York, N.Y.) p. 86.

CHAPTER
5

This chapter summarizes briefly the findings of the study and devotes major attention to an interpretation of their effect upon community planning for mental health aftercare services.

The Findings

In sum, here is what the study found:

1. Over 10,500 patients are released from Pennsylvania's state mental hospitals each year; nine out of ten of these patients require one or more aftercare services when they leave.

2. Facilities and services are available to meet 97% of the aftercare recommendations for released patients; the mental hospitals themselves carry on an extensive aftercare service program providing one-half of these services.

3. The major aftercare service recommendations for patients fall within the medical-social triad of medication, counseling, and psychotherapy; vocational and resocialization services constitute a minor proportion.

4. About one out of four released patients are rehospitalized within one year; the most frequent factor precipitat-

ing patients' return is inability to cope with stressful situations. Over one-third of the patients are returned for this reason.

5. A little less than half (44%) of returned patients might have avoided rehospitalization if aftercare services had been available and used. For over half (56%), their rehospitalization would have occurred regardless of utilization of available aftercare services.

6. Over 40% of the reasons aftercare services are not used is because patients refuse the service; an additional 40% of the reasons have to do with either the nonavailability of services or breakdown in operations of the service system.

7. There is evidence to indicate that, as available aftercare services are used more frequently by released patients, fewer patients will require rehospitalization.

The study findings may also be useful to help guide the development of aftercare programs in any statewide Comprehensive Mental Health Plan. The study data are assembled and classified by planning regions so that mental health authorities can use this profile of aftercare needs and services for planning regional and local programs. Thus, in addition to answering the research questions raised by the study on a statewide basis, results of this study provide *for each planning region* the following guideline information which could be used in estimating present and future aftercare needs:

a. The number of patients who will be released from state mental hospitals to the region.

b. The distribution of their aftercare needs.

c. Their living arrangements and employability status.

d. The availability of services to meet the recommended needs.

e. The number of patients who can be expected to be rehospitalized.

48

f. The primary reasons for rehospitalization, with special reference to the effect of the provision of aftercare services on rehospitalization.

g. The nature of the utilization problem and its relationship to the rate of return.

THE HYPOTHESES OF THIS STUDY*

As a result of the study, the following hypotheses are accepted:

1. Eighty-five percent of all patients leaving state hospitals will require one or more aftercare services.

2. The higher the rate of utilization of available aftercare services, the lower the rate of return.

The following hypotheses are rejected:

1. Reemployment and resocialization services constitute the principal aftercare needs of patients at discharge.

2. (a) Aftercare facilities are insufficient in number throughout the state.

(b) They are primarily available in the large metropolitan areas of the state.

3. The state return percentage will approximate the national return percentage.

4. The most frequent cause of patients' return to hospital within one year after leaving is the lack of aftercare services.

HYPOTHESES FOR FURTHER TESTING

Additional hypotheses growing out of the study and suggested for further testing can be stated briefly as follows:

1. Patients with available economic resources are more likely to be released than those who are medically indigent.

2. Patients who will be living with their own families are more likely to be released than those who do not have families to return to in the community.

*See Appendix: I

3. A substantial proportion of patients remain in state mental hospitals for economic and family reasons rather than for psychiatric reasons.

4. Hospital staffs tend to recommend aftercare services for released patients on the basis of the known availability of such services.

5. State-supported community psychiatric clinics have a policy and practice of rejecting for service released patients from state mental hospitals.

6. A carefully planned program of foster home finding and placement would provide a substantial resource for appropriate living arrangements for patients now being kept in state hospitals who could be released.

7. The reemployment rate of released patients could be substantially increased through the expansion of the present counseling and job placement program of the State Bureau of Vocational Rehabilitation.

8. Investigation will reveal that certain hospitals have developed workable and effective techniques for active involvement of private physicians, churches, and selected community agencies in the provision of aftercare services for released patients; these techniques can be identified, described, and articulated for use in all regions.

9. The rate of return of released patients from state hospitals is affected by the degree of hospital overcrowding and shortages of hospital staff; the rate of return will go up as overcrowding and staff shortages go down.

10. There is a direct relationship between low rate of utilization of aftercare services and released patients' failure to seek employment while out of hospital; these two factors are pivotal for community tenure.

In light of the results of this study a number of modifications are indicated in the Comprehensive Mental Health Plan (see Appendix: III):

1. It is doubtful that "a network of sheltered work-

shops and employment centers and a regional vocational training center" should be established in each region. This proposal was based on the assumption that about half the patients released from state hospitals would be candidates for employment and that a significant section of them would require special or sheltered types of occupation. The data reveal that less than 20% of the total patients released might have unmet needs in the vocational field. Only a fraction of these would require sheltered employment. Therefore, a network of such services is certainly not indicated.

2. It is doubtful also whether "early attention should be given to establishing halfway houses or other types of residential facilities for discharged or 'on-leave' patients." Rather, the data indicate that in the development of new types of facilities, additional consideration might be given to the day treatment center which is only partially "residential." The findings indicate that there is growing recognition of the day treatment center as a resource for more of the specialized, "sheltered" aftercare requirements of released patients.

With respect to the need for additional foster family care, this is not supported by the findings. However, it is suggested that efforts be made to determine the feasibility of expansion of this program, which may make it possible for some patients now retained in hospital to be released.

3. The proposal that "local citizens' groups be asked to sponsor social clubs for former patients in those areas where no such clubs exist" is also of doubtful merit. Only 6% of the recommendations for released patients called for referral of patients to such clubs; 98% of the recommendations could be fulfilled through available resources, according to hospital staff.

4. While it may be true that "current research indicates that public health nurses can assist patients . . . in home-care programs," the results of this study indicate that

51

Pennsylvania state mental hospital staffs are not using this resource. Only 83 of a total of 16,824 recommendations (0.5%) were made to public health nursing organizations for study patients. Implementing this proposal would require a radical change in practice which could come about only if there was conviction on the part of hospital staffs that public health nursing could be effective in this regard.

5. One of the crucial aftercare services is counseling. This is defined in a number of ways. In the final report of the Comprehensive Plan, it is denoted as a service provided by social agencies. In the Aftercare Study, it is defined as a service which can be rendered by a social agency, by a psychiatric clinic, by clergy, or by mental hospital staff. (See Appendix: *Schedules.*) In the working definition of the Task Force Report, it is classified under the social services, along with casework and group work services, assistance with living arrangements, income maintenance, and other health and welfare services. Counseling is differentiated from resocialization services, although it falls within the same general category. Since this service is so pivotal, both as to the number of times it was recommended for study patients upon release (19%) and the number of times it was cited as an aftercare service which could have prevented patients' return (15%), the Comprehensive Plan should revise, redefine and, in general, explicate the counseling concept and its application.

Further investigation of the precise meaning and practice of regulation of medication is indicated also. Statements of two released patients interviewed in the Allegheny County study are revealing. One of them said: "I decided to cut the number of pills in half—they last twice as long and I can't see any difference." Another patient, who apparently had not been seeing a physician while taking medication, was asked about this. He averred that he can always tell when he's had enough drugs. He stops taking them when his thumbs begin to get numb.

6. Finally, the emphasis of the aftercare recommendations of the Comprehensive Mental Health Plan must be redirected to the core needs of patients—namely, medication, counseling, and psychotherapy, which constitute approximately 75% of the needs of the released patient and 60% of the services which could have prevented patient's return. The Plan's recommendations are focused primarily on resocialization, sheltered living, and employment services.

Two Proposals Are Supported

While the results of this study suggest changes in the aftercare proposals of the Comprehensive Plan, two proposals of the Plan are strongly supported by the results of this study. The first has to do with the community-based model of services. The second has to do with personnel requirements.

1. The key to the development of community-based services for released patients from state hospitals is the relationship between hospital and community. The results of this study show that these are, from the point of view of delivery of aftercare services, two separate worlds. Only in the use of hometown physicians for supervision and regulation of medication has there been any substantial working partnership between hospital and community developed in the interests of the released patient. This is true not only in small communities but also in the large metropolitan areas where there is a plethora of health and welfare services which could, if properly mobilized, provide the needed aftercare service programs and thus help the released patient find roots once again in his community. It should be kept in mind that no research has established that community-based services are more effective than hospital-based services for the seriously mentally ill.

This study raises the question of the respective values of hospital and community auspices for aftercare services.

53

It would seem of considerable importance that certain specific steps be undertaken to test out best ways of making the maximum use of both hospital and community services *in a coordinated and cooperative program,* since both may have significant roles to play. This is particularly so if the Plan's major recommendation that each community mental health center develop an extensive aftercare program is carried forward.

2. The Plan recommends that high priority be given to the development of training and recruitment of three types of staff to perform specialized aftercare functions: (a) community organization specialist; (b) counselor or caseworker; (c) rehabilitation worker. These functions are rooted to social work knowledge and skill. The social worker, whether hospital or community based, is trained to help the patient mobilize all his resources to deal with his personal and social needs. The focus of the social worker's effort is helping the patient to uncover his own strengths —his "abilities" rather than "disabilities"—to meet and cope with the obstacles which stand in the way of his reintegration into community living. The problem of utilization of available aftercare services is particularly suited to social work intervention. The social worker can be the vital link between client and community—between the patient and the services he needs.

An extraordinary effort will be needed to mobilize the social work personnel required to do the job. It should be noted that the present social worker complement of the state hospitals meets only one-third the minimum (see Appendix: IV) standards of the American Psychiatric Association.

The critical question of utilization has been dealt with in this study; there still remains a lot to be learned about it. However, one thing is very clear; without some built-in and carefully designed assistance, released patients who need aftercare services most will not get them. The Plan's strong emphasis on the development of specialized personnel, particularly the second category of counselor or caseworker defined as the person who "attaches himself" to the patient, is strongly supported by the findings of this study.

It has been said that only one who has lived through the experience can really know or grasp the nature of serious mental illness. Some talented and creative people have written about their own experiences, from Beers to Sartre. All refer to the critical moments of coming out of the depths into the real world once again, and what this rapid and radical change in milieu presents to the patient who is trying to reestablish himself. There is no mistaking that what most ex-patients seek is a human relationship which can be trusted to help provide the support and the continuing link until the ways of the "new world" are relearned. Beers said that what the mentally ill need is a friend. In the Allegheny County survey, a psychiatrist observed: "for these people, trying to get squared around back home, there's no substitute for a warm body."

While creative and talented persons give the description in depth of the despair and horror of disabling mental illness, one of the released patients interviewed in the Allegheny County put his finger on why an aftercare program has to be welded with "human" glue. This man was released after a fairly long period of hospitalization. He came back to his hometown—a big city. He found many things strange and frightening, including the public transportation system. He tells of trying to make his first appointment at the clinic:

> "I told a man I'd pay him to go with me. Somehow we missed connections and I had to go alone. I got on the first streetcar that came along. After I'd ridden a long time, I found out I was going the wrong way. Later, when I had to change streetcars, I didn't want to ask for a piece of paper, so I just kept putting money in the box. Must have spent two dollars."

55

No aftercare program can be fully productive unless there is full recognition and understanding of the nature of the clientele to be served and the special problems it has in availing itself of services. Skilled personnel "attached to the patient" is one way of dealing with the special problems.

It should be repeated that the purpose of providing aftercare services is not solely to prevent rehospitalization. This may be a side effect of considerable importance. But the primary motivation for providing and helping released patients use aftercare services is that these persons need and, hopefully, can be helped to use these services. This is a goal per se, and attempting to gild it over with purposes and goals of secondary importance only obscures the main target—the patient and his struggle to deal with his problems.

This is not to say that the secondary values should be overlooked. Helping a released patient become, once again, a full citizen, participating in community life with the duties and responsibilities which full citizenship implies, may indeed be community psychiatry of the highest order. Its psychotherapeutic effect for the patient cannot be measured.

This "view from the bridge" would indicate that perhaps there are individual and social goals in aftercare which, when they coalesce, are the mark of achievement.

PART
II

The Planning Process

CHAPTER
6

PRELUDE TO PLANNING

In 1955, a joint resolution of the 84th Congress became Public Law 182, popularly known as the "Mental Health Study Act of 1955." This Act created the Joint Commission on Mental Illness and Health, charged with providing the Congress with "an objective, thorough and nationwide evaluation of the human and economic problems of mental illness"(1).

A series of monographs was prepared under the direction of the Joint Commission. A final report, entitled "Action for Mental Health," was published in 1961(2). Its recommendations gave the impetus for a national effort in comprehensive planning for community mental health services.

A principal contribution of the Joint Commission was the development of guidelines for a reorganization of care and treatment methods for the mentally ill. The recommendations were based on the idea of care and treatment facilities at the local or regional level through the establishment of mental health centers to provide *comprehensive* community mental health programs in the local community. The *prevention* of disability is stressed. But with the

59

onset of illness, prompt diagnosis, effective early treatment, aftercare, and rehabilitation of the patient are em-
phasized. In short, community mental health programs are
intended to meet the total spectrum of patient need and to
be available as needed, whether over long or short, continuous or intermittent periods of time, and within, if possible,
the patient's own community(3).

The Community Mental Health Centers Act of 1963
(4) represented a major step toward implementation of the
Joint Commission's recommendations. Among other provisions, this Act authorized funds for the construction of community mental health centers. In 1965 the Act was amended,
appropriating federal funds to be used for personnel.

A list of the type of services in a community mental
health center program includes:

a. Diagnostic and evaluation services
b. Inpatient services for acute and chronic patients
c. Part-time hospitalization (day care and night care
   programs)
d. Outpatient and clinical service
e. Around-the-clock emergency service
f. Rehabilitation and aftercare services
g. Consultation services to other agencies and institutions
h. Public information and education services
i. Research, evaluation, coordination, and planning
   services
j. Training of personnel

As a prerequisite for the establishment of these centers, Congress appropriated funds in fiscal 1963 and 1964
for grants to the states to prepare statewide plans for comprehensive mental health programs.

THE PENNSYLVANIA PLANNING PROJECT

In the latter part of 1962, when it became clear that
federal planning funds for a state study might become

available, a Pennsylvania planning-steering committee was set up by the Commissioner of Mental Health. Representatives of Pennsylvania Mental Health, Inc., the Pennsylvania Association for Retarded Children, health and welfare councils in Pennsylvania, the Pennsylvania Medical Society, the Pennsylvania Psychiatric Society, and the six medical schools in Pennsylvania developed a first draft of a plan. This draft was reviewed by advisory committees of the Office of Mental Health, the State Board of Public Welfare, and the commissioners of various program offices of the Department of Public Welfare. In addition, members of the Senate and House of Representatives of the General Assembly, representatives of the Pennsylvania AFL-CIO, and representatives of the State Planning Board, including business and industry members, reviewed the draft proposal.

In June 1963, the Office of Mental Health of the Department of Public Welfare submitted a final draft to the National Institute of Mental Health of the U.S. Public Health Service, Department of Health, Education, and Welfare. Within three weeks, the proposal was accepted and a grant of $398,600 was made available to the Commonwealth of Pennsylvania for a comprehensive mental health planning study, to be completed by September 1965.

THE TASK FORCES

According to the design of the study, two principal efforts were undertaken. The first was the establishment of task forces, composed of professional persons whose assignment was "to deliberate and report on specific professional content within their fields of competence." In total, there were 42 task forces(5), each consisting of a chairman and approximately 10 members, to examine specific areas of mental health program. One Task Force was assigned the problem of aftercare. The report of this Task Force provided the hypotheses for this study of aftercare.

61

Each Task Force was guided by a general outline to assist in the preparation of its final report or "position paper." The outline included: (a) a working definition of the specific Task Force title, (b) description of resources, (c) a statement of needs, (d) evaluation of resources (relation of resources to needs), (e) problem areas (selection of at least two key areas of greatest concern), (f) research in the area of interest, and (g) evaluation and recommendations.

THE REGIONAL COMMITTEES

The second broad dimension of the plan was the regionalization of the state and the establishment of regional committees. Eight planning regions were established. The criteria for the selection of the eight planning regions were: (a) mental health service areas sufficiently large to support comprehensive mental health centers and residential care, as well as containing clearly delineated communities in which coordinated day care, rehabilitation, and training programs could be planned; (b) natural service areas based upon known utilization of health, hospital, and welfare services; (c) administrative and planning requirements necessary for the collection of data, local planning activity, and future implementation; (d) population and socioeconomic factors; (e) comprehensive planning characteristics.

Guides to the selection of planning regions took into consideration the Commonwealth's identification of hospital needs, based on the "Hill-Burton" requirements for aid to hospitals, the service areas of the Department of Health, service areas for state mental hospitals, and schools for the mentally retarded.

A regional committee was appointed in each of the eight regions, composed of representatives from the following bodies: county commissioners, United Fund and community councils, county medical societies, state hospital superintendents, general hospital administrators, mental health and mental retardation associations, public health officers, professional associations (psychiatrists, psychologists, nurses, social workers, lawyers, and judges) and five members selected at large. The assignment given to each regional committee was:

1. Develop an inventory of prior planning recommendations made in their regions.

2. Develop an inventory of services and site visitation programs of facilities in their regions.

3. Hold "gatekeeper" meetings to receive testimony from groups and individuals such as lawyers, police, educators, judges, etc.

4. Hold public meetings throughout the region to receive testimony from citizens in general.

5. Confer with the citizen voluntary organizations— i.e., representatives of Pennsylvania Mental Health, Inc. and the Pennsylvania Association for Retarded Children.

On the basis of its activity, each regional committee was assigned the task of producing a proposed "regional plan"(6). The central project staff had the task of developing the eight regional plans and the reports of the Task Forces into a statewide body of knowledge as the basis for a Commonwealth Comprehensive Mental Health Plan.

In December 1965, the Comprehensive Mental Health Plan of the Commonwealth of Pennsylvania(7) was completed, approved by the appropriate committees, and transmitted to the Governor. After review by the administration and by legislative leaders, legislation to implement the plan was drawn up, introduced, and passed in the 1966 session of the Pennsylvania General Assembly.

REFERENCES

1. U.S. Congress, Public Law 182, 84th Congress, First Session, Res. 256.

2. *Op. cit.*

3. U.S. Congress, House, Subcommittee of the Committee on Interstate and Foreign Commerce, *Hearings,* H.R. 3688, 88th Congress, First Session, March 26, 27, and 28, 1963.

4. U.S. Congress, Public Law 88-164, Title 11, October, 1963.

5. For a summary of highlights of Task Force Reports: Pennsylvania Mental Health, Inc., Philadelphia, Pa. "What Every MHA Director Should Know About the Task Force Reports."

6. For a summary of highlights of Regional Committee Reports: Pennsylvania Mental Health, Inc. Philadelphia, Pa. "What Every MHA Director Should Know About the Regional Committee Reports."

7. Commonwealth of Pennsylvania. "The Comprehensive Mental Health Plan." Clifford J. Bodarky, Ed. (Health and Welfare Building, Harrisburg, Pa.) 1965.

CHAPTER
7

THE PLANNING REGIONS

A brief description of the eight planning regions(1), and the state mental hospitals which serve them, provides a background for analysis of the aftercare problem by regions.

Since 1955 there has been an upward improvement trend in the state mental hospitals as measured by per diem per patient expenditures and by ratios of staff to patients. The average daily expenditure per patient in 1955 was $2.60; the average per diem per patient expenditure in 1964 was $5.80. It is estimated that approximately half of this increase was due to rising costs and approximately half for "improvement." In 1955, the staff complement for the state hospitals was approximately 9,000 persons; in 1964, it was approximately 12,500. During this same period, there was a gradual decrease in the total number of patients in residence. In June 1955, there were 40,920 in-hospital patients; in June 1964, there were 36,795 in-hospital patients. During the same period, there was an increase in admissions to the state hospitals. In 1955, there were 7,708 admissions and in 1964 there were 10,704 admissions (see Table 1).

In short, the experience in Pennsylvania reflects the national trends in these categories.

TABLE 1
PATIENTS RESIDING IN STATE MENTAL HOSPITALS OR ON LEAVE, AND NUMBER OF PATIENTS PER 100,000 POPULATION IN PENNSYLVANIA: 1955 TO 1964

Year	In Hospital	On Leave of Absence	Total	Number per 100,000 Population
1955	40,920	8,277	49,197	451
1956	39,947	9,266	49,213	448
1957	39,717	10,100	49,817	450
1958	39,507	10,239	49,746	446
1959	39,347	10,583	49,930	444
1960	38,668	11,647	50,315	445
1961	38,096	12,961	51,057	448
1962	37,478	14,042	51,520	449
1963	37,205	15,106	52,311	452
1964	36,811	16,456	53,267	456

Source: Pennsylvania Statistical Abstract, 1964-65, Pennsylvania Department of Public Welfare, Office of Program Research and Statistics, February 1965, p. 141.

Despite the progress, however, Pennsylvania's state hospitals continue to be plagued with staff shortages and overcrowded conditions. In 1964, for example, the eighteen state mental hospitals employed about 8,500 *treatment* staff; meeting minimum personnel standards of the American Psychiatric Association would require 3,500 additional treatment staff(2). In short, the key staff is 40% below the minimum for proper staff-to-patient ratios. In some categories of personnel the deficit is more critical than in others. The APA standard calls for 347 social workers; only 170 social work positions are authorized. (See pps. 143-149 for individual hospital personnel complements.)

THE PLANNING REGIONS

REGION I includes ten counties in Southwestern Pennsylvania, with a total population of 3,057,421 (1964 estimate): Allegheny, Armstrong, Beaver, Butler, Fayette,

FIGURE 1
PLANNING REGIONS

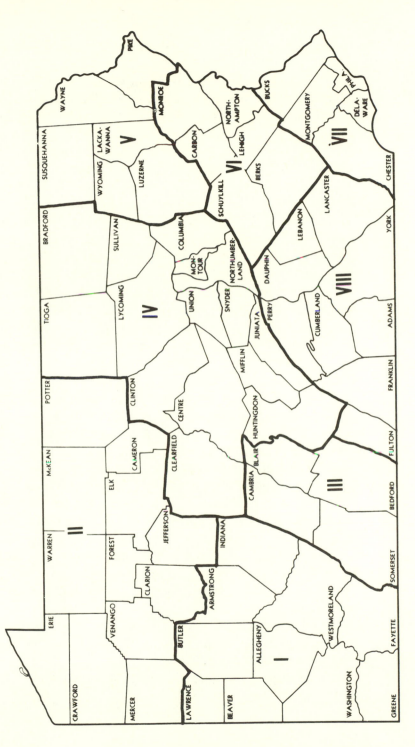
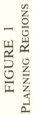

Greene, Indiana, Lawrence, Washington, and Westmoreland.

Allegheny, a second-class county, includes 129 incorporated civil divisions and the city of Pittsburgh, the second largest in the state. The county also has three third-class cities: Clairton, Duquesne, and McKeesport.

The counties range in population from Greene, with a low of 37,000, to Allegheny with approximately 1,660,000.

The range in economic status is broad, including Fayette County, with the highest unemployment rate of all the counties in the state, to the active mill areas of Butler and Beaver counties, where there is a labor shortage, to Pittsburgh, which is the center of one of the world's largest steel-producing areas.

Population projections indicate that there will be decreases in population in Greene, Fayette, Indiana, and Armstrong; moderate increases (up to 10%) in Allegheny, Washington, Westmoreland, and Lawrence, and large increases (ranging from 10 to more than 53%) in Butler and Beaver.

There is a major concentration of health and welfare services and facilities in the city of Pittsburgh. There is an uneven distribution of health and welfare services in the rest of the region, with some notable exceptions. Kittanning, in Armstrong County, for example, has developed mental health facilities which are highly adequate in proportion to the population, while other counties have no psychiatric facilities except what is offered by the state hospital.

The region is served by four state mental hospitals: Dixmont, Mayview, Torrance, and Woodville.

Dixmont State Hospital serves Beaver and Lawrence counties, with a total population of 337,995. The hospital has a rated capacity of 706 and, in June 1964, it had a resident population of patients numbering 924. The percentage occupancy was 131.1%.

The hospital provides a limited outpatient service for

68

discharged patients. In June 1964, 38 patients were receiving service.

Mayview State Hospital serves the city of Pittsburgh, with a total population of approximately 900,000 people. The hospital has a rated capacity of 2,684.

In June 1964, the number of resident patients in the hospital was 2,902. The percentage occupancy was 108%.

The hospital provides an outpatient service for discharged patients. In June 1964, 1,029 patients received service.

Torrance State Hospital serves Armstrong, Butler, Greene, Indiana, Westmoreland, and Washington counties, with a total population of approximately 903,025.

In June 1964, the number of resident patients in the hospital was 3,062. The percentage occupancy was 154.4%.

The hospital provides an outpatient service for discharged patients. In June 1964, 44 patients received service.

Woodville State Hospital serves a portion of Allegheny County, with a total population of approximately 774,165 people. The hospital has a rated capacity of 2,137.

In June 1964, the number of resident patients in the hospital was 2,496. The percentage occupancy was 117.6%.

The hospital provides no outpatient service for discharged patients.

REGION II includes thirteen counties in Northwestern Pennsylvania, with a total population of 870,731: Cameron, Clarion, Clearfield, Crawford, Elk, Erie, Forest, Jefferson, McKean, Mercer, Potter, Venango, and Warren.

Erie County, with the Commonwealth's third largest city, Erie, has an estimated 1964 population of 264,046. Forest County, with an estimated 1964 population of 4,455, is the smallest in the region and in the state.

Crawford County, with a population of 77,728, and

Mercer County, with a population of 134,231, are the other two counties of the thirteen next to Erie in size, which can be looked at from a planning point of view as unitary. The other counties can be described in clusters for this purpose.

Crawford County is a sixth-class county, with Meadville as its principal population center.

Mercer County has two principal centers of population, with approximately 500,000 persons located in the Shenango Valley towns of Sharon, Farrell, and Sharpsville. The balance are located in outlying communities: Greenville, Mercer, Grove City, and small rural communities and farms.

Venango, Forest, and Clarion counties have an approximate population of 106,642 persons. Of this number, nearly two-thirds are located in Venango County, principally in the Oil City-Franklin area. Forest County has two principal communities: Tionesta (800) and Marienville (800). Clarion County has one principal community: Clarion, with a population of slightly under 5,000.

Cameron, Elk, Jefferson, and Potter counties have an approximate population of 108,533. Cameron has one principal community: Emporium, with a population of 3,397. The principal communities are St. Marys (8,065) and Ridgway (6,387).

Jefferson, the largest of the four, has the principal towns of Brookville (4,620) and Punxsutawney (8,805).

Potter County's principal community is Coudersport (2,889).

Warren and McKean counties have a population of 101,323. Approximately one-half of the population is in the major towns of Warren, Bradford, and Kane. The Allegheny National Forest occupies approximately 50% of the land area in Warren and over one-third of McKean County, resulting in a widely scattered population outside the three major towns.

Erie County has a fairly well-developed group of health and welfare services. A skeletal health and welfare establishment exists in Mercer and Crawford counties. One of the unique developments in this region is the Ridgway Area Psychiatric Center, a state-supported outpatient service located in Elk County and serving—in addition to Elk —Cameron, Potter, McKean, Clearfield, Jefferson, and Forest counties.

The region is served by *Warren State Hospital*. The hospital has a rated capacity of 2,028.

In June 1964, the number of resident patients in the hospital was 2,470. The percentage occupancy was 122.4%.

The hospital provides an outpatient service for discharged patients. In June 1964, 194 patients received service.

REGION III includes six counties, with a total population of 496,852 persons: Bedford, Blair, Cambria, Fulton, Huntingdon, and Somerset.

The two principal population centers are the city of Johnstown, in Cambria County, a fourth-class county, and the city of Altoona, in Blair County, a fifth-class county.

Approximately 50% (100,000) of the population of Cambria County live in the city of Johnstown. In Blair County, about 50% (70,000) live in Altoona. These two centers have fairly well-developed health and welfare services, including some psychiatric clinical services. The other counties in the area have no psychiatric services except those provided by the state hospitals.

The region is served by two state hospitals—Hollidaysburg and Somerset.

Hollidaysburg State Hospital has a rated capacity of 787.

In June 1964, the number of resident patients in the hospital was 870. The percentage occupancy was 112.2%.

71

The hospital provides an outpatient service for discharged patients. In June 1964, 183 patients received service.

Somerset State Hospital has rated capacity of 702.

In June 1964, the number of resident patients in the hospital was 682. The percentage occupancy was 97.7%.

The hospital provides an outpatient service for discharged patients. In June 1964, 114 patients received service.

REGION IV includes twelve counties, with a total population of 614,825: Bradford, Centre, Clinton, Columbia, Lycoming, Mifflin, Montour, Northumberland, Snyder, Sullivan, Tioga, and Union.

This is a sparsely populated region, with two principal population centers: Lycoming County, with a population of 109,367, including the city of Williamsport, and Northumberland County, with a population of 104,138, with the cities of Sunbury and Shamokin.

About half the region is Appalachian plateau; the rest is mountainous. Transportation is a major problem; bus and rail service is negligible, and airports are remote and subject to weather hazards.

There are some unique features in the region which should be taken into account in the planning of services. In the complex of Bradford and Sullivan counties, while no community facilities exist, the presence of an outstanding medical institution in the city of Sayre, Bradford County— the Robert Packer Hospital—has the makings of a community mental health center with perhaps a branch development in the town of Towanda.

In Columbia County, with the centers of population, Bloomsburg and Berwick, family counseling services have been developed and the potential for the development of community mental health center programs is promising.

In Union County, the presence of the Geisinger Medical Center, a nationally recognized institution with a developing psychiatric service, also has potential for the development of community mental health programs.

Centre County, the home of Pennsylvania State University, could provide a resource for the development of community services in that area of the region.

The above examples are by way of illustrating the possibilities of overcoming the severe handicaps presented by the geography and population dispersement characteristic of this region.

The region is served by *Danville State Hospital.* The hospital has a rated capacity of 2,472.

In June 1964, the number of resident patients in the hospital was 2,251. The percentage occupancy was 91.6%.

The hospital provides an outpatient service for discharged patients. In June 1964, 741 patients received service.

REGION V includes six counties, with a total population of 676,472 persons: Lackawanna, Luzerne, Pike, Susquehanna, Wayne, and Wyoming.

About one-third of the region's population lives within a 25-mile (elliptical) circle of Wilkes-Barre and Scranton, the two large metropolitan areas. Scranton, in Lackawanna County, and Wilkes-Barre, in Luzerne County, were once the centers of coal mining. This industry is now a shadow of its former self.

Since the end of World War II, concerted efforts to establish heavy and light manufacturing have had considerable success and provided increasing opportunities for employment in the area.

Agriculture and agricultural products predominate in Wayne, Pike, Susquehanna, and Wyoming Counties.

Virtually all of the health and welfare services are located in Scranton and Wilkes-Barre and this is where a large majority of the region's people seek services. Trans-

73

portation facilities throughout the region are quite adequate and offer good intercity and intercounty transportation.

The area was hard hit during the economic depression of the 1930's. The outward migration of families and particularly the young adult population was high and continued through 1960. There is evidence that this emigration is leveling off with the upsurge of new industry, extensive construction of superhighways, and the development of large tracts of land for commercial and residential use.

Health and welfare services in the Scranton-Wilkes-Barre area are relatively well developed. The fact that the region has been a "depressed area" for over 30 years has induced the Commonwealth and local public and private groups to concentrate on the provision of these services. The potential for developing community mental health programs to serve the region, therefore, exists in considerable measure.

The region is served by two state mental hospitals: *Clarks Summit,* in Lackawanna County, and *Retreat,* in Luzerne County.

Clarks Summit has a rated capacity of 1,328.

In June 1964, the number of resident patients in the hospital was 1,217. The percentage occupancy was 92.5%.

The hospital provides an outpatient service for discharged patients. In June 1964, 605 patients received service.

Retreat State Hospital has a rated capacity of 582.

In June 1964, the number of resident patients in the hospital was 886. The percentage occupancy was 132.5%.

The hospital provides no outpatient service for discharged patients.

REGION VI includes six counties, with a population of 987,969: Berks, Carbon, Lehigh, Monroe, Northampton, and Schuylkill.

The region includes the relatively prosperous Lehigh

Valley communities of Allentown, Bethlehem, and Easton. Other population centers are Reading, in Berks County, Stroudsburg, in Monroe County, and Pottsville, in Schuylkill County.

A large variety of heavy and light manufacturing industries can be found in the major cities. However, Schuylkill and Carbon counties, where mining was the major industry, are only beginning to recover industrially with the influx of other types of economic activities. Transportation facilities are excellent throughout the region.

Allentown, in Lehigh County, has a population of slightly over 100,000 and is the center for extensive health and welfare services in the Lehigh Valley. Its links with Bethlehem and Easton, in Northampton County, have been established through planning and coordinating agencies in health, welfare, and recreation. On the other hand, Carbon and Schuylkill counties have a limited number of services and are considered two counties in this region requiring special attention.

The region is served by two state mental hospitals: Allentown, in Lehigh County, and Wernersville, in Berks County.

Allentown State Hospital has a rated capacity of 1,430.

In June 1964, the number of resident patients in the hospital was 1,530. The percentage occupancy was 111.6%.

The hospital provides an outpatient service for discharged patients. In June 1964, 521 patients received service.

Wernersville State Hospital has a rated capacity of 1,666.

In June 1964, the number of resident patients in the hospital was 1,657. The percentage occupancy was 98.8%.

The hospital provides an outpatient service for discharged patients. In June 1964, 56 patients received service.

75

REGION VII includes Bucks, Chester, Delaware, Montgomery, and Philadelphia counties, with a total population of 3,769,243. At the heart of the region is the city of Philadelphia and its metropolitan area which, for planning and other purposes, includes the entire region.

No brief comment would suffice to describe this region. In general, the region is the most well developed with respect to mental health facilities. There is great variety and abundance of health and welfare services. Paralleling this wealth of resources is the high incidence of need and the judgment has been made that the services to meet them are inadequate.

The area is served by four state mental hospitals: Philadelphia, Norristown, Haverford, and Embreeville.

Philadelphia State Hospital has a rated capacity of 4,937.

In June 1964, the number of resident patients in the hospital was 6,353. The percentage occupancy was 128.3%.

The hospital provides an outpatient service for discharged patients. In June 1964, 1,772 patients received service.

Norristown State Hospital has a rated capacity of 3,790.

In June 1964, the number of resident patients in the hospital was 3,845. The percentage occupancy was 100.9%.

The hospital provides an outpatient service for discharged patients. In June 1964, 890 patients received service.

Haverford State Hospital has a rated capacity of 550.

In June 1964, the number of resident patients in the hospital was 546. The percentage occupancy was 99%.

The hospital provides an outpatient service for discharged patients. In June 1964, 595 patients received service.

Embreeville State Hospital has a rated capacity of 1,325.

In June 1964, the number of resident patients in the hospital was 1,011. The percentage occupancy was 79.6%.

The hospital does not provide outpatient service for discharged patients.

REGION VIII includes nine counties with a total population of 1,203,137: Adams, Cumberland, Dauphin, Franklin, Juniata, Lancaster, Lebanon, Perry, and York.

The counties in this region, with the exception of Perry and Fulton, represent one of the most prosperous areas of the state economically, yet, despite a remarkable industrial expansion since World War II, the region remains a principal agricultural center of the state.

The most populous counties are Dauphin, Lancaster, and York, each with its principal cities of Harrisburg, Lancaster, and York. A fourth major urban center is the city of Lebanon in Lebanon County.

There was loss of population by the four large cities in the region from 1950 to 1960 amounting to 7.7%, although the increase in the overall population of the region was 17%. The greatest growth has been in the urban fringe of the major cities, amounting to 162% in Lancaster, 146% in York, and 62% in the Harrisburg (Dauphin) urban fringe.

There has been extensive development of health and welfare services, including mental health, in the three principal cities. These population centers are linked with good highways and the suburban semirural and rural areas of the region are within relatively good access of the health and welfare services. The noncity areas are characterized by a diversity of farming production, and employment in agriculture is nearly two-and-a-half times that of the state average.

The region is served by *Harrisburg State Hospital* which has a rated capacity of 2,099.

In June 1964, the number of resident patients in the

hospital was 2,374. The percentage occupancy was 112.2%.

The hospital provides an outpatient service for discharged patients. In June 1964, 146 patients received service.

As can be seen, the planning regions and the state mental hospitals within them are in some ways a study in variations and contrasts. This is a reflection, of course, of the character of the state as a whole. For example, the average density of population in Pennsylvania is about 250 persons per square mile. But this varies from 16,000 persons per square mile in Philadelphia to about 16 persons per square mile in the north-central portion of the state(3).

Thus, planning for services must reflect the variations and special requirements of each service and planning area. The next chapter provides the data on which regional aftercare programs can be designed.

REFERENCES

1. Data sources: Department of Internal Affairs, 7th Annual Edition, Commonwealth of Pennsylvania. *Pennsylvania Statistical Abstract: 1964-65.* (Harrisburg, Pa.) "Regional Committee Reports," Comprehensive Mental Health Plan, Office of Mental Health, Department of Public Welfare (Harrisburg, Pa.).

2. Pennsylvania Mental Health, Inc. "A Profile of the Eighteen State Mental Hospitals in Pennsylvania," (Philadelphia, Pa.) February 1965.

3. For a comprehensive statement of state characteristics, from which much of this summary is taken, see "The Comprehensive Mental Health Plan," (Harrisburg, Pa.) pp. 64-68; and, *Pennsylvania Statistical Abstract, op. cit.*

CHAPTER
8

A BASIS FOR PLANNING

The data, tabulations, and commentary which follow, include aftercare needs of discharged patients, availability of services to meet these needs, return rates and precipitating factors, and the utilization of aftercare services, by regions.

AFTERCARE NEEDS

In Region I, which includes the metropolitan area of Pittsburgh, there were 1,849 releases, or 17% of the total state releases. During the study period, 104 of the study patients were released from the hospital more than once. Of the total releases, 136 were judged not to require any aftercare services. This is 7.3% of the total releases in the region. For the remainder, there was a total of 2,920 recommendations for specific aftercare services, indicating that a substantial number of patients required more than one type of aftercare service (Table 1).

Living arrangements for the study patients in Region I leaving the hospitals show that approximately 9% will live alone, 30% with spouse, and 45% with other relatives. Approximately 3% will live with nonrelatives or in foster

TABLE 1

NUMBER OF TIMES SELECTED AFTERCARE SERVICES
RECOMMENDED FOR STUDY PATIENTS IN REGION I

Aftercare Services	Number	Percentage	State Percentage
TOTAL	2,920	100.0%	100.0%
Regulation of medication	1,155	39.4	45.0
Counseling services	644	22.0	18.9
Public Assistance	259	8.8	3.8
Vocational rehabilitation	257	8.8	6.2
Resocialization services	175	6.0	3.6
Psychotherapy	165	5.6	13.0
Alcoholics Anonymous	140	4.7	4.9
Sheltered living	53	1.8	2.6
Public Health Nursing	29	0.9	0.5
Day treatment services	2	—	0.2
Other	41	1.3	1.3

TABLE 1A

STUDY PATIENTS IN REGION I WHO WILL BE
ENTERING LABOR MARKET, JOB READINESS,
EMPLOYABILITY STATUS AT TIME OF RELEASE

	Number	Percentage	State Percentage
TOTAL	926	100.0%	100.0%
Returning to former position:			
Yes	217	23.4	29.3
No	677	73.1	63.7
No report	32	3.5	7.0
Job readiness:			
Poor	68	7.3	5.0
Fair	547	59.0	52.3
Good	270	29.2	39.0
No report	41	4.5	3.7

family care. Approximately 12% were transferred to other institutional settings—nursing homes, county homes, and other institutions.

Data on job readiness and employability status of study patients released in Region I, as shown in Table 1A, indicate that approximately one-half (926) of the released patients will enter the labor market. Of these patients, 217, or less than 25%, will be returning to former positions.

Of the total 1,849 releases, 923, or 50% will not be entering the labor market. Distribution of reasons for patients not entering the labor market is shown in Table 1B.

TABLE 1B
REASONS FOR STUDY PATIENTS IN REGION I
NOT ENTERING LABOR MARKET

Reasons	Number	Percentage	State Percentage
TOTAL	923	100.0%	100.0%
Household duties	406	44.0	38.5
Physical or mental disability	193	20.6	25.0
Age	122	13.2	15.5
Institutionalized after leaving hospital	91	9.8	8.7
Inability to adjust to employment	63	6.2	3.9
No report	48	5.2	8.4

In Region II, which includes the city of Erie, there were 906 releases, or 8.5% of total state releases. Thirty-nine of the study patients were released from the hospital more than once during the study period. Of the total releases, 56 were judged not to require any aftercare services. This is 6% of the total of 1,044 recommendations for specific aftercare services, indicating that some patients required more than one type of service (Table 2).

TABLE 2
NUMBER OF TIMES SELECTED AFTERCARE RECOMMENDED
FOR STUDY PATIENTS IN REGION II

Aftercare	Number	Percentage	State Percentage
TOTAL	1,044	100.0%	100.0%
Regulation of medication	442	42.3	45.0
Psychotherapy	181	17.3	13.0
Counseling services	99	9.4	18.9
Alcoholics Anonymous	91	8.7	4.9
Vocational rehabilitation	85	8.1	6.2
Resocialization services	61	5.8	3.6
Sheltered living	43	4.1	2.6
Public Assistance	25	2.3	3.8
Day treatment services	1	—	0.2
Public Health Nursing	0	—	0.5
Other	16	1.5	1.3

TABLE 2A
STUDY PATIENTS IN REGION II WHO WILL BE
ENTERING LABOR MARKET, JOB READINESS,
EMPLOYABILITY STATUS AT TIME OF RELEASE

	Number	Percentage	State Percentage
TOTAL	383	100.0%	100.0%
Returning to former position:			
Yes	128	33.6	29.3
No	191	50.0	63.7
No report	63	16.4	7.0
Job readiness:			
Poor	11	2.8	5.0
Fair	158	41.2	52.3
Good	198	51.9	39.0
No report	16	4.1	3.7

Living arrangements for the study patients leaving the hospitals show that approximately 3% will live alone,

83

45% with spouse, and 40% with other relatives. Approximately 2% will live with nonrelatives or in foster family care. Approximately 10% were transferred to other institutional settings—nursing homes, county homes, and other institutions.

Data on job readiness and employability status of study patients at the time of release, as shown in Table 2A, indicate that, of the total 906 releases, 383, or 42.2%, will enter the labor market. Of this number, 128, or 36.6%, will be returning to former positions.

Of the total 906 releases, 523, or 37.8%, will not be entering the labor market. Distribution of reasons for not entering the labor market is shown in Table 2B.

TABLE 2B
REASONS FOR STUDY PATIENTS IN
REGION II NOT ENTERING LABOR MARKET

Reasons	Number	Percentage	State Percentage
TOTAL	523	100.0%	100.0%
Household duties	288	55.2	38.5
Age	113	21.6	15.5
Physical or mental disability	68	13.0	25.0
Institutionalized after leaving hospital	42	8.0	8.7
Inability to adjust to employment	0	—	3.9
No report	12	2.2	8.4

In Region III, which includes the cities of Johnstown and Altoona, there were 696 releases, or 6.5% of the total state releases. Thirty-six of the study patients were released from the hospital more than once during the study period. Of this number, 50 were judged not to require any aftercare services. This is 7% of the total releases in the region. For the remainder, there was a total of 1,173 recommenda-

tions for specific aftercare services, indicating that a majority of patients required more than one type of service
(Table 3).

TABLE 3

NUMBER OF TIMES SELECTED AFTERCARE RECOMMENDED
FOR STUDY PATIENTS IN REGION III

Aftercare	Number	Percentage	State Percentage
TOTAL	1,173	100.0%	100.0%
Regulation of medication	509	43.4	45.0
Counseling services	283	24.1	18.9
Vocational rehabilitation	106	9.0	6.2
Psychotherapy	71	6.0	13.0
Sheltered living	59	5.0	2.6
Alcoholics Anonymous	57	4.8	4.9
Public Assistance	42	3.5	3.8
Resocialization services	32	2.7	3.6
Day treatment services	4	0.3	0.2
Public Health Nursing	0	0.0	0.5
Other	10	0.9	1.3

Living arrangements for the study patients leaving the
hospitals show that approximately 5% will live alone,
40% with spouse, and 40% with other relatives. Approximately 4% will live with nonrelatives or in foster family
care. Approximately 8% were transferred to other institutional settings—nursing homes, county homes, and other
institutions.

Data on job readiness and employability status of
study patients at the time of release, as shown in Table 3A,
indicate that, of the total 696 releases, 255, or 36.6%, will
enter the labor market. Of these, 87, or 34%, will be returning to their former positions.

Distribution of reasons for patients not entering the
labor market is shown in Table 3B.

TABLE 3A
STUDY PATIENTS IN REGION III WHO WILL BE
ENTERING LABOR MARKET, JOB READINESS,
EMPLOYABILITY STATUS AT TIME OF RELEASE

	Number	Percentage	State Percentage
TOTAL	255	100.0%	100.0%
Returning to former position:			
Yes	87	34.0	29.3
No	166	65.0	63.7
No report	2	1.0	7.0
Job readiness:			
Poor	21	8.0	5.0
Fair	150	60.0	52.3
Good	82	31.0	39.0
No report	2	1.0	3.7

In Region IV, which includes the city of Williamsport, there were 799 releases, or 7% of the total state releases. Twenty-nine of the study patients were released from the

TABLE 3B
REASONS FOR STUDY PATIENTS IN REGION III
NOT ENTERING LABOR MARKET

Reasons	Number	Percentage	State Percentage
TOTAL	441	100.0%	100.0%
Household duties	183	41.5	38.5
Physical or mental disability	98	22.3	25.0
Age	89	20.2	15.5
Institutionalized after leaving hospital	25	5.6	8.7
Inability to adjust to employment	10	2.2	3.9
No report	36	8.2	8.4

TABLE 4
NUMBER OF TIMES SELECTED AFTERCARE RECOMMENDED
FOR STUDY PATIENTS IN REGION IV

Aftercare	Number	Percentage	State Percentage
TOTAL	1,428	100.0%	100.0%
Counseling services	472	24.6	18.9
Regulation of medication	453	22.7	45.0
Alcoholics Anonymous	150	10.6	4.9
Psychotherapy	128	9.0	13.0
Resocialization services	101	7.7	3.6
Vocational rehabilitation	58	4.0	6.2
Sheltered living	40	2.8	2.6
Public Assistance	16	1.1	3.8
Public Health Nursing	3	—	0.5
Day treatment services	1	—	0.2
Other	6	0.4	1.3

hospital more than once during the study period. Of the total releases, 26 were judged not to require any aftercare services. This represents 3% of the total releases in the region. For the remainder, there was a total of 1,428 recommendations for specific aftercare services, indicating that a majority of patients required more than one type of service (Table 4).

Living arrangements for the study patients leaving the hospitals show that approximately 11% will live alone, 40% with spouse, and 35% with other relatives. Less than 2% will live with nonrelatives or in foster family care. Approximately 10% were transferred to other institutional settings—nursing homes, county homes, and other institutions.

Data on job readiness and employability status of study patients at the time of release, as shown in Table 4A, indicate that 331, or 41.5% of the total 799 releases, will enter the labor market. Of these, 171, or 51.6%, will return to their former positions.

TABLE 4A
STUDY PATIENTS IN REGION IV WHO WILL BE
ENTERING LABOR MARKET, JOB READINESS,
EMPLOYABILITY STATUS AT TIME OF RELEASE

	Number	Percentage	State Percentage
TOTAL	331	100.0%	100.0%
Returning to former position:			
Yes	171	51.6	29.3
No	159	48.4	63.7
No report	1	—	7.0
Job readiness:			
Poor	1	—	5.0
Fair	120	36.3	52.3
Good	209	—	39.0
No report	1	—	3.7

Of the total 799 releases, 468, or 58.5%, will not enter the labor market. Distribution of reasons for patients not entering labor market is shown in Table 4B.

TABLE 4B
REASONS FOR STUDY PATIENTS IN REGION IV
NOT ENTERING LABOR MARKET

Reasons	Number	Percentage	State Percentage
TOTAL	468	100.0%	100.0%
Household duties	205	43.9	38.5
Inability to adjust to employment	106	22.7	3.9
Age	61	12.8	15.5
Physical or mental disability	60	12.8	25.0
Institutionalized after leaving hospital	30	6.2	8.7
No report	9	1.8	8.4

In Region V, which includes the cities of Wilkes-Barre and Scranton, there were 584 releases, or 5% of the total state releases. Thirty-eight of the study patients were released from the hospital more than once during the study period. Of the total releases, 173 were judged not to require any aftercare services. This represents 30% of the total releases in the region. For the remainder, there was a total of 1,039 recommendations for specific aftercare services, indicating that a majority of patients required more than one type of service (Table 5).

TABLE 5

NUMBER OF TIMES SELECTED AFTERCARE RECOMMENDED
FOR STUDY PATIENTS IN REGION V

	Number	Percentage	State Percentage
TOTAL	1,039	100.0%	100.0%
Regulation of medication	422	40.6	45.0
Counseling services	235	22.6	18.9
Vocational rehabilitation	107	10.3	6.2
Psychotherapy	89	8.5	13.0
Resocialization services	70	6.7	3.6
Public Assistance	50	4.8	3.8
Sheltered living	26	2.5	2.6
Alcoholics Anonymous	18	1.7	4.9
Public Health Nursing	1	—	0.5
Day treatment services	1	—	0.2
Other	20	1.9	1.3

Living arrangements for the study patients leaving the hospitals show that approximately 6% will live alone, 37% with spouse, and 38% with other relatives. Approximately 3% will live with nonrelatives or in foster family care. Approximately 8% were transferred to other institutional settings—nursing homes, county homes, and other institutions.

89

Data on job readiness and employability status of study patients at the time of release are indicated in Table 5A. A total of 252, or 43.1%, are expected to enter the

---

TABLE 5A

STUDY PATIENTS IN REGION V WHO WILL BE
ENTERING LABOR MARKET, JOB READINESS,
EMPLOYABILITY STATUS AT TIME OF RELEASE

	Number	Percentage	State Percentage
TOTAL	252	100.0%	100.0%
Returning to former position:			
Yes	84	33.0	29.3
No	157	62.4	63.7
No report	11	4.5	7.0
Job readiness:			
Poor	28	11.2	5.0
Fair	127	50.4	52.3
Good	86	33.8	39.0
No report	11	4.5	3.7

TABLE 5B

REASONS FOR STUDY PATIENTS IN
REGION V NOT ENTERING LABOR MARKET

	Number	Percentage	State Percentage
TOTAL	332	100.0%	100.0%
Household duties	163	49.0	38.5
Age	62	18.4	15.5
Physical or mental disability	59	17.4	25.0
Institutionalized after leaving hospital	23	7.1	8.7
Inability to adjust to employment	1	—	3.9
No report	24	7.1	8.4

labor market. Eighty-four, or 33%, of these were returning to former positions.

Distribution of reasons for study patients not entering the labor market in Region V upon release is shown in Table 5B.

In Region VI, which includes the cities of Allentown, Bethlehem, Easton, and Reading, there were 783 releases, or 7% of the total state releases. Forty-two of the study patients were released from the hospital more than once during the study period. Of this number, 73 were judged not to require any aftercare services. This represents 10% of the total releases in the region. For the remainder, there was a total of 1,705 recommendations for specific after-care services, indicating that a majority of patients required more than one type of service (Table 6).

TABLE 6

NUMBER OF TIMES SELECTED AFTERCARE
RECOMMENDED FOR STUDY PATIENTS IN REGION VI

Aftercare	Number	Percentage	State Percentage
TOTAL	1,705	100.0%	100.0%
Regulation of medication	632	37.0	45.0
Counseling services	401	23.5	18.9
Psychotherapy	312	18.3	13.0
Resocialization services	85	4.9	3.6
Vocational rehabilitation	79	4.6	6.2
Public Assistance	52	3.0	3.8
Alcoholics Anonymous	39	2.2	4.9
Sheltered living	31	1.8	2.6
Day treatment services	28	1.5	0.2
Public Health Nursing	14	0.8	0.5
Other	32	1.8	1.3

Living arrangements for the study patients leaving the hospitals show that approximately 6% will live alone, 40% with spouse, and 40% with other relatives. Approximately 3% will live with nonrelatives or in foster family care. Approximately 7% were transferred to other institutional settings—nursing homes, county homes, and other institutions.

TABLE 6A

STUDY PATIENTS IN REGION VI WHO WILL BE
ENTERING LABOR MARKET, JOB READINESS,
EMPLOYABILITY STATUS AT TIME OF RELEASE

	Number	Percentage	State Percentage
TOTAL	373	100.0%	100.0%
Returning to former position:			
Yes	126	34.0	29.3
No	227	60.0	63.7
No report	20	6.0	7.0
Job readiness:			
Poor	16	4.5	5.0
Fair	184	50.0	52.3
Good	157	41.0	39.0
No report	16	4.5	3.7

TABLE 6B

REASONS FOR STUDY PATIENTS IN
REGION VI NOT ENTERING LABOR MARKET

Reasons	Number	Percentage	State Percentage
TOTAL	410	100.0%	100.0%
Household duties	135	33.0	38.5
Physical or mental disability	127	31.0	25.0
Age	78	19.0	15.5
Institutionalized after leaving hospital	41	10.0	8.7
Inability to adjust to employment	8	2.0	3.9
No report	21	5.0	8.4

Data on job readiness and employability status of study patients at the time of release are shown in Table 6A. A total of 373, or 47.6%, were expected to enter the labor market; 126, or 34%, were expected to return to their former positions.

Distribution of reasons for patients not entering the labor market upon release are shown in Table 6B. Of the study patients, 410, or 52.4% of releases, were not expected to enter the labor market.

In Region VII, which includes the metropolitan area of Philadelphia, there were 4,363 releases, or 40% of the total state releases. Of the study patients, 303 were released from the hospital more than once during the study period. Of the total releases, 487 were judged not to require any aftercare services. This represents 11% of the total releases in the region. For the remainder, there was a total of 6,420 recommendations for specific aftercare services, indicating that a substantial number of patients required more than one type of service (Table 7).

TABLE 7

NUMBER OF TIMES SELECTED AFTERCARE
RECOMMENDED FOR STUDY PATIENTS IN REGION VII

	Number	Percentage	State Percentage
TOTAL	6,420	100.0%	100.0%
Regulation of medication	3,449	53.6	45.0
Psychotherapy	1,225	19.0	13.0
Counseling services	744	11.5	18.9
Vocational rehabilitation	267	4.1	6.2
Alcoholics Anonymous	167	2.5	4.9
Public Assistance	157	2.4	3.8
Sheltered living	147	2.2	2.6
Resocialization services	80	1.2	3.6
Public Health Nursing	28	0.4	0.5
Day treatment services	11	0.1	0.2
Other	145	2.2	1.3

Living arrangements for the study patients leaving the hospitals show that approximately 9% will live alone, 30% with spouse, and 42% with other relatives. Approximately 7% will live with nonrelatives or in foster family care. Approximately 8% were transferred to other institutional settings—nursing homes, county homes, and other institutions.

Data on job readiness and employability status of study patients at the time of release, as shown in Table 7A, indicate that 2,272, or 51.9% of the study patients in Region VII were expected to enter the labor market. Of these, 586, or 26%, will be returning to former positions.

TABLE 7A

STUDY PATIENTS IN REGION VII WHO WILL BE
ENTERING LABOR MARKET, JOB READINESS,
EMPLOYABILITY STATUS AT TIME OF RELEASE

	Number	Percentage	State Percentage
TOTAL	2,272	100.0%	100.0%
Returning to former position:			
Yes	586	26.0	29.3
No	1,478	65.0	63.7
No report	208	9.0	7.0
Job readiness:			
Poor	101	4.5	5.0
Fair	1,137	50.0	52.3
Good	942	41.5	39.0
No report	92	4.0	3.7

Distribution of reasons for patients not entering the labor market upon release is shown in Table 7B. Of the total 436 releases, 2,091, or 48.1%, are not expected to enter the labor market.

In Region VIII, which includes the cities of Harrisburg, Lancaster, and York, there were 806 releases, or

TABLE 7B

REASONS FOR STUDY PATIENTS IN REGION VII
NOT ENTERING LABOR MARKET

Reasons	Number	Percentage	State Percentage
TOTAL	2,091	100.0%	100.0%
Physical or mental disability	731	35.0	25.0
Household duties	643	30.7	38.5
Age	284	13.6	15.5
Institutionalized after leaving hospital	206	9.8	8.7
Inability to adjust to employment	33	1.6	3.9
No report	194	9.2	8.4

7.5% of the total state releases. Forty-two of the study patients were released from the hospital more than once during the study period. Of the total releases, 136 were judged not to require any aftercare services. This represents

TABLE 8

NUMBER OF TIMES SELECTED AFTERCARE
RECOMMENDED FOR STUDY PATIENTS IN REGION VIII

Aftercare	Number	Percentage	State Percentage
TOTAL	1,095	100.0%	100.0%
Regulation of medication	512	46.7	45.0
Counseling services	302	27.5	18.9
Vocational rehabilitation	89	8.1	6.2
Sheltered living	42	3.8	2.6
Public Assistance	35	3.2	3.8
Alcoholics Anonymous	26	2.3	4.9
Psychotherapy	21	1.9	13.0
Resocialization services	10	0.9	3.6
Public Health Nursing	8	0.7	0.5
Day treatment services	1	—	0.2
Other	50	4.5	1.3

17% of the total releases in the region. For the remainder, there was a total of 1,095 recommendations for specific aftercare services, indicating that a substantial number of patients required more than one type of service (Table 8).

Living arrangements for the study patients leaving the hospitals show that approximately 6% will live alone, 40% with spouse, and 37% with other relatives. Approximately 4% will live with nonrelatives or in foster family care. Approximately 9% were transferred to other institutional settings—nursing homes, county homes, and other institutions.

TABLE 8A

STUDY PATIENTS IN REGION VIII WHO WILL BE
ENTERING LABOR MARKET, JOB READINESS,
EMPLOYABILITY STATUS AT TIME OF RELEASE

	Number	Percentage	State Percentage
TOTAL	398	100.0%	100.0%
Returning to former position:			
Yes	126	31.7	29.3
No	244	61.3	63.7
No report	28	7.0	7.0
Job readiness:			
Poor	12	3.1	5.0
Fair	239	60.0	52.3
Good	123	30.8	39.0
No report	24	6.1	3.7

Data on job readiness and employability status of study patients at the time of release, as shown in Table 8A, indicate that, of the total 806 releases, 398, or 49.3%, were expected to enter the labor market. Of these, 126, or 31.7%, were expected to return to their former positions.

Distribution of reasons for patients not entering the

labor market upon release is shown in Table 8B. Of the total 806 releases, 408, or 50.7% are not expected to enter the labor market.

In the eight planning regions, the findings on the aftercare problem are indicative of a number of variations from the statewide profile.

1. In Region I, the combined aftercare services—medication, counseling, and psychotherapy—constitute 67% of all recommendations as compared to the 75%

TABLE 8B

REASONS FOR STUDY PATIENTS IN REGION VIII
NOT ENTERING LABOR MARKET

	Number	Percentage	State Percentage
TOTAL	408	100.0%	100.0%
Household duties	164	40.0	38.5
Physical or mental disability	88	21.5	25.0
Age	84	20.8	15.5
Institutionalized after leaving hospital	36	9.0	8.7
Inability to adjust to employment	2	0.5	3.9
No report	34	9.0	8.4

state proportion. Recommendations for psychotherapy account, for the most part, for this divergence; it ranks sixth (5.6%) in Region I, as compared to the state rank of three (13.0%). Psychotherapy recommendations are replaced in the rank order in Region I by public assistance recommendations. The statewide proportion for public assistance is 3.8%; in Region I it is 8.8%.

Twice as many released patients (12%) were transferred to other institutions in Region I as is the case in the statewide proportion (5.8%).

In Region I, 92.5% of study patients were recommended for one or more aftercare services, as compared to the statewide proportion of 89.5%.

2. In Region II, 85% of released patients will live with spouse or other relatives, compared to the 75% statewide proportion. Only 3% will live alone, as compared to the statewide proportion of 7.6%. Ten percent were transferred to other institutions, as compared to the statewide proportion of 5.8%.

This is one of two regions in which more than half (51.9%) of released patients were considered good employment risks.

Ninety-four percent of study patients were recommended for one or more aftercare services in Region II, as compared to the statewide proportion of 89.5%.

3. In Region III, recommendations for sheltered living arrangements for released patients were approximately twice the statewide proportion—5%, as compared to 2.6%.

Only 36.6% of total releases are expected to enter the labor market, as compared to the statewide proportion of 47.3%.

Ninety-three percent of study patients were recommended for one or more aftercare services in Region III, as compared to the statewide proportion of 89.5%.

4. In Region IV, counseling services replace regulation of medication as the most frequent aftercare recommendation for released patients. This is the only region in which this displacement occurs—i.e., that regulation of medication recommendations do not lead the list. It is also significant to note that the combined aftercare service recommendations—medication, psychotherapy, and counseling—constitute 56.3% of the recommendations, as compared to the statewide proportion of 75%.

Recommendations for Alcoholics Anonymous repre-

98

sented 10.6% of aftercare recommendations, as compared to the statewide proportion of 4.9%.

The proportion of public assistance recommendations is the lowest of all regions—1.1%—as compared to the statewide proportion of 3.6%.

More than half (51.6%) of those expected to enter the labor market on release will be returning to their former positions. This compares to the statewide proportion of 29.3%. Of those patients entering the labor market, 53.7% are considered good employment risks, as compared to the statewide proportion of 39%; this is the second of two regions in which this is a finding.

Ninety-seven percent of study patients were recommended for one or more aftercare services in Region IV, as compared to the statewide proportion of 89.5%.

5. In Region V, the striking finding is that only 70% of releases were judged to require one or more aftercare services. This compares to the statewide proportion of 89.5%. This is the lowest percentage of all regions.

In Region V, the combined aftercare services of vocational rehabilitation and resocialization constitute 17% of the recommendations. This compares to the statewide proportion of 9.8%.

6. In Region VI, the findings reflect the statewide picture, with no significant variations.

7. In Region VII, the findings represent 40% of the aftercare needs of all study patients and influence the statewide proportions accordingly.

Eighty percent of all released patients (3,499) in Region VII received a "regulation of medication" recommendation. The combined aftercare services—medication, psychotherapy, and counseling—constituted 85% of the total recommendations for aftercare services. This compares with the statewide proportion of 75%.

The combined vocational rehabilitation and resocial-

TABLE 9

Availability of Regulation of Medication Recommended for Study Patients; Regional Provisions for Service

	Regions							
	I	II	III	IV	V	VI	VII	VIII
Is service available?								
Yes	1,155	440	507	453	421	631	3,436	512
No	0	2	2	0	1	1	3	0
Who will provide service?								
Hospital	658	77	151	355	235	377	2,036	174
Private physician	470	349	354	97	177	230	1,345	334
Community clinic	25	14	2	1	0	17	30	1
No report	2	0	0	0	9	7	25	3

TABLE 10
COUNSELING AVAILABLE FOR STUDY PATIENTS
AND REGIONAL PROVISIONS FOR SERVICE

				Regions				
	I	II	III	IV	V	VI	VII	VIII
Is service available?								
Yes	626	56	237	437	222	392	732	300
No	13	43	46	35	12	7	10	1
Who will provide service?								
Hospital	555	20	189	330	196	295	556	260
Private physician	26	11	5	3	11	27	57	5
Community clinic	5	4	5	5	0	11	26	14
Social agency	18	11	19	63	3	32	47	14
Clergy	8	4	6	2	3	3	7	1
Other	12	3	13	33	6	17	21	4
No report	2	3	0	1	3	7	19	2

TABLE 11

Availability of Psychotherapy Recommended for Study Patients and Regional Provisions for Service

				Regions				
	I	II	III	IV	V	VI	VII	VIII
Is service available?								
Yes	162	135	51	128	24	311	1,196	18
No	3	45	20	0	65	1	20	2
Who will provide service?								
Hospital	124	86	22	117	12	270	837	6
Private physician	30	27	22	9	8	27	284	11
Community clinic	7	22	7	2	0	11	40	0
No report	1	0	0	0	2	2	26	1

TABLE 12

AVAILABILITY OF VOCATIONAL REHABILITATION RECOMMENDED FOR STUDY PATIENTS AND REGIONAL PROVISIONS FOR SERVICE

	Regions							
	I	II	III	IV	V	VI	VII	VIII
Is service available?								
Yes	257	84	101	58	104	78	262	89
No	0	1	5	0	3	0	3	0
Who will provide service?								
Bureau of Voc. Rehabilitation	154	83	93	58	102	66	230	85
Other	4	1	7	0	2	6	28	2
No report	0	0	1	0	0	6	6	2

TABLE 13

Availability of Resocialization Recommended for Study Patients and Regional Provisions for Service

	I	II	III	IV	V	VI	VII	VIII
				Regions				
Is service available?								
Yes	164	19	9	101	67	40	70	9
No	10	42	23	0	3	35	10	1
Who will provide service?								
Ex-patients' club	137	17	2	1	43	13	45	1
Community center	5	0	2	4	5	18	9	3
Church	15	1	0	96	6	4	4	0
Other	6	1	5	0	10	5	11	5

TABLE 14

Availability of Sheltered Living Recommended for Study Patients and Regional Provisions for Service

	Regions							
---	I	II	III	IV	V	VI	VII	VIII
Is service available?								
Yes	50	37	51	40	25	30	147	38
No	3	6	9	0	1	1	0	1
Who will provide service?								
Family care	11	2	22	19	2	3	41	4
Nursing home	9	20	6	3	4	12	32	21
County home	6	11	12	9	7	8	3	4
Halfway house	2	0	2	1	0	1	19	0
Rooming house	4	1	1	1	2	0	15	0
Other	16	2	8	7	8	6	33	9

TABLE 15

AVAILABILITY OF SELECTED SERVICES RECOMMENDED FOR STUDY PATIENTS AND REGIONAL PROVISIONS FOR SERVICE

	Regions							
	I	II	III	IV	V	VI	VII	VIII
Day treatment center:								
Is service available?								
Yes	1	0	0	1	1	2	11	0
No	1	1	4	0	0	26	0	0
Alcoholics Anonymous:								
Is service available?								
Yes	137	90	47	149	18	37	166	24
No	1	1	10	1	0	2	0	2
VNA or public health nurse:								
Is service available?								
Yes	29	0	0	3	1	14	28	8
No	0	0	0	0	0	0	0	0
Public Assistance	259	25	42	16	50	52	157	35
Other services	126	22	23	81	29	70	301	37

TABLE 16
STUDY PATIENTS RETURNED TO HOSPITAL, BY REGIONS, DURING 12-MONTH PERIOD

Region	Releases	Did Not Return for 12 Months	Returned During 12 Months	Return Rate by Percentage of Releases
Statewide	10,786	8,005	2,781	25.7
I	1,849	1,403	445	24.0
II	906	669	237	26.1
III	696	510	186	26.7
IV	799	643	156	19.5
V	584	441	143	24.4
VI	783	593	190	24.5
VII	4,363	3,166	1,198	27.3
VIII	806	582	224	27.9

TABLE 17
FACTORS WHICH PRIMARILY PRECIPITATED PATIENTS' RETURNS IN REGION I

Factors	Number	Percentage	State Percentage
TOTAL	492	100.0%	100.0%
Inability to cope with stressful situations	172	34.9	35.0
Refused or discontinued medication	72	14.6	13.7
Negative family environment	48	9.7	9.4
Excessive drinking	45	9.1	6.9
Premature release	23	4.6	6.5
Other environmental problems	19	3.9	6.1
Recurrence of previous symptoms	9	1.8	5.6
Different symptoms from previous illness	12	2.4	2.7
Other	31	6.3	5.7
No report	61	12.3	8.3

107

ization recommendations totaled 5.3%, compared to the statewide proportion of 9.8%.

The public assistance recommendations (2.4%) also fell behind the statewide proportion (3.8%).

A lower proportion of employable released patients in Region VII will be returning to their former positions— 26% as compared to the statewide proportion of 30%. A higher proportion of study patients in Region VII will not be entering the labor market because of physical and mental disability (35%), as compared to the statewide proportion of 25%.

8. In Region VIII, the findings reflect the statewide picture, with little significant variation, except in respect to the number of study patients requiring aftercare services. The proportion of study patients in Region VIII judged to need such services is 83%, as compared to the statewide proportion of 89.5%.

While there are, as shown above, variations among the planning regions with respect to the aftercare service needs of study patients, one critical area of agreement does stand out. The social and vocational services are not considered as pressing needs. This is in marked contrast to the general concern expressed in professional, governmental, and citizens' groups with the problems of developing such aftercare services as halfway houses, sheltered workshops, vocational rehabilitation and resocialization programs. This concern is spelled out in clear and unmistakable terms as high priority requirements for aftercare planning in the final report of the Comprehensive Mental Health Plan.

The findings of this part of the study would suggest that, in the judgment of the hospital staffs, there is considerable doubt that the extent and nature of social and vocational needs of patients who leave would warrant high priority attention. While it may be premature to conclude that the recommendations of the Comprehensive Mental Health Plan should be altered to correspond to the findings reported thus far in this study, it is entirely proper to conclude that a vital question has been opened up for further inquiry.

AVAILABILITY OF AFTERCARE SERVICES

The availability of recommended aftercare services for study patients in each region, and the facilities to which referrals were made for providing these services, are shown in Tables 9 to 15.

In Region I, there was a total of 2,920 aftercare recommendations for study patients, for which services for 2,840 were judged to be available. This is an availability rate of 97.2%.

In Region II, there was a total of 1,044 aftercare recommendations, for which services for 896 were judged to be available. This is an availability rate of 85.7%.

TABLE 18

FACTORS WHICH PRIMARILY PRECIPITATED
PATIENTS' RETURNS IN REGION II

Factors	Number	Percentage	State Percentage
TOTAL	238	100.0%	100.0%
Inability to cope with stressful situations	34	14.3	35.0
Refused or discontinued medication	16	6.7	13.7
Negative family environment	17	6.7	9.4
Excessive drinking	27	11.3	6.9
Premature release	17	6.7	6.5
Other environmental problems	6	2.5	6.1
Recurrence of previous symptoms	58	20.3	5.6
Different symptoms from previous illness	10	4.2	2.7
Other	6	2.9	5.7
No report	47	19.8	8.3

TABLE 19
FACTORS WHICH PRIMARILY PRECIPITATED
PATIENTS' RETURNS IN REGION III

Factors	Number	Percentage	State Percentage
TOTAL	197	100.0%	100.0%
Inability to cope with stressful situations	60	30.5	35.0
Refused or discontinued medication	31	15.7	13.7
Negative family environment	32	15.7	9.4
Excessive drinking	4	2.0	6.9
Premature release	18	9.2	6.5
Other environmental problems	22	11.2	6.1
Recurrence of previous symptoms	5	2.1	5.6
Different symptoms from previous illness	—	—	2.7
Other	14	7.2	5.7
No report	11	5.6	8.3

In Region III, there was a total of 1,173 aftercare recommendations, for which services for 1,045 were judged to be available. This is an availability rate of 89.0%.

In Region IV, there was a total of 1,428 aftercare recommendations, for which services for 1,392 were judged to be available. This is an availability rate of 97.4%.

In Region V, there was a total of 1,039 aftercare recommendations, for which services for 954 were judged to be available. This is an availability rate of 91.8%.

In Region VI, there was a total of 1,705 aftercare recommendations, for which services for 1,632 were judged to be available. This is an availability rate of 95.7%.

In Region VII, there was a total of 6,420 aftercare recommendations, for which services for 6,374 were judged to be available. This is an availability rate of 99.2%.

In Region VIII, there was a total of 1,095 aftercare recommendations, for which services for 1,087 were judged to be available. This is an availability rate of 99.2%.

The range in availability rate is from the low of 85.7% in Region II to the 99.2% in Regions VII and VIII.

While Philadelphia, one of the two large metropolitan areas, is in Region VII, its availability rate is matched by Region VIII, and approached by the availability rate of Region IV, both nonmetropolitan areas.

Region I, which includes Pittsburgh, the second large metropolitan area, is matched by the availability rate of Region IV, and is below that of Region VIII, a nonmetropolitan area.

TABLE 20

FACTORS WHICH PRIMARILY PRECIPITATED
PATIENTS' RETURNS IN REGION IV

Factors	Number	Percentage	State Percentage
TOTAL	166	100.0%	100.0%
Inability to cope with stressful situations	57	34.3	35.0
Refused or discontinued medication	12	7.2	13.7
Negative family environment	10	6.0	9.4
Excessive drinking	18	10.8	6.9
Premature release	9	5.4	6.5
Other environmental problems	7	4.2	6.1
Recurrence of previous symptoms	43	25.9	5.6
Different symptoms from previous illness	6	3.6	2.7
Other	3	1.8	5.7
No report	1	0.6	8.3

TABLE 21
FACTORS WHICH PRIMARILY PRECIPITATED
PATIENTS RETURNS IN REGION V

Factors	Number	Percentage	State Percentage
TOTAL	160	100.0%	100.0%
Inability to cope with stressful situations	67	41.7	35.0
Refused or discontinued medication	34	21.2	13.7
Negative family environment	14	8.8	9.4
Excessive drinking	7	4.4	6.9
Premature release	4	2.5	6.5
Other environmental problems	9	5.6	6.1
Recurrence of previous symptoms	4	2.5	5.6
Different symptoms from previous illness	4	2.5	2.7
Other	9	5.6	5.7
No report	8	5.0	8.3

All in all, the differential in availability rates between regions is small.

A number of unique characteristics in the various regions with respect to the available facilities used to provide recommended aftercare services for study patients may be worthy of note:

1. In Regions II, III, and VIII, for example, private physicians are used extensively in providing regulation of medication services to released patients. In these regions, the private physicians' services exceed by far the services given by the state hospitals in the region for this category of aftercare. In Region II, there were 349 recommendations to private physicians, as compared to the 77 provided by the state hospital. In Region III, there were 354 refer-

rals made to private physicians, as compared to the hospital's service to 151. In Region VIII, there were 334 referrals for this service to private physicians, as compared to the 174 served by the hospital. In all other regions, the hospitals provided a majority of the services in this category.

2. In Regions III and VIII, again, the referrals to private physicians constituted a substantial proportion of psychotherapy recommendations for the study patients, while in all other regions an overwhelming percentage of these services were provided by the hospital itself.

3. In Region IV, the churches provided resocialization services for 96 study patients. Throughout the state, there were only 126 instances of a church providing this service.

TABLE 22
FACTORS WHICH PRIMARILY PRECIPITATED
PATIENTS' RETURNS IN REGION VI

Factors	Number	Percentage	State Percentage
TOTAL	210	100.0%	100.0%
Inability to cope with stressful situations	85	40.5	35.0
Refused or discontinued medication	18	8.6	13.7
Negative family environment	11	5.2	9.4
Excessive drinking	14	6.6	6.9
Premature release	6	2.9	6.5
Other environmental problems	6	2.9	6.1
Recurrence of previous symptoms	23	10.9	5.6
Different symptoms from previous illness	8	3.8	2.7
Other	33	15.7	5.7
No report	6	2.9	8.3

TABLE 23
FACTORS WHICH PRIMARILY PRECIPITATED
PATIENTS' RETURNS IN REGION VII

Factors	Number	Percentage	State Percentage
TOTAL	1,304	100.0%	100.0%
Inability to cope with stressful situations	503	38.6	35.0
Refused or discontinued medication	203	15.5	13.7
Negative family environment	110	8.4	9.4
Excessive drinking	71	5.4	6.9
Premature release	114	8.5	6.5
Other environmental problems	96	8.3	6.1
Recurrence of previous symptoms	21	1.5	5.6
Different symptoms from previous illness	34	2.6	2.7
Other	51	3.9	5.7
No report	101	8.3	8.3

This is such a deviation from the general practice that it might be worth discovering how and under what conditions this unique situation has come about.

In sum, the data indicate that, regionally, the availability of aftercare services to meet recommendations made by hospitals staffs for study patients does not present a problem.

RETURN RATES, PRECIPITATING FACTORS

Table 16 shows the rate of return, by regions, indicating that Region IV had the lowest rate (19.5%) and Region VIII had the highest rate (27.9%).

It may be of interest to review, briefly, what the judgments were with respect to aftercare needs of all patients who were released (Chapter 4) in Region IV, with the lowest return rate (19.5%), and in Region VIII, with the highest return rate (27.9%).

Region IV, for example, with the lowest return rate, is the only region which places counseling first in frequency distribution of recommended aftercare services for its released patients. The region has other unique characteristics. The triad of medication, counseling, and psychotherapy constituted 56% of all recommended aftercare services, as compared to the state percentage of 75%. More than twice the state percentage of its released patients were referred to Alcoholics Anonymous. Region IV also referred the lowest proportion of its released patients for public assistance— 1.1%, as compared to 3.6%. It should be noted that in Region IV 97% of released patients were referred for one

TABLE 24

FACTORS WHICH PRIMARILY PRECIPITATED
PATIENTS' RETURNS IN REGION VIII

Factors	Number	Percentage	State Percentage
TOTAL	242	100.0%	100.0%
Inability to cope with stressful situations	77	31.8	35.0
Refused or discontinued medication	28	11.6	13.7
Negative family environment	41	17.0	9.4
Excessive drinking	22	9.0	6.7
Premature release	6	2.4	6.5
Other environmental problems	18	7.5	6.1
Recurrence of previous symptoms	6	2.4	5.6
Different symptoms from previous illness	6	2.4	2.7
Other	22	9.0	5.7
No report	16	6.6	8.3

TABLE 25
AFTERCARE SERVICES WHICH COULD HAVE PREVENTED
PATIENTS' RETURN TO HOSPITAL IN REGION I

Aftercare	Number	Percentage	State Percentage
TOTAL	314	100.0%	100.0%
Regulation of medication	78	25.0	28.3
Counseling	52	16.6	14.5
Psychotherapy	28	8.9	13.1
Day treatment center	26	8.3	10.8
Alcoholics Anonymous	35	11.1	7.4
Sheltered living arrangements	22	7.0	7.4
Vocational rehabilitation	20	6.9	5.7
Resocialization	29	8.6	5.5
Other	18	6.8	5.7
No report	6	2.0	—

or more aftercare services, as compared to the state percentage of 89.5%. More than half (51.6%) of released patients who were expected to enter the labor market were returning to former positions. This compares to the state percentage of 29.3%. It is significant that hospital staff judged that 53.7% of these patients were considered good employment risks, as compared to the statewide proportion of 39%.

On the other hand, Region VIII, with the highest return rate, reflects the statewide proportions in all respects, with the exception that 83% of its released patients were referred for aftercare, as compared to the state percentage of 89.5%.

As can be seen from Table 25, the findings in Region I with respect to aftercare service needs of returned patients while out of hospital correspond in general to the statewide findings on this point.

A few striking features appear in the data on this question. These deserve brief preliminary mention. In the first instance, it was to be expected that the recurrence of previous symptoms would constitute a major factor in returns. It is commonly held that many of the illnesses, particularly the psychoses and functional disorders, are recurrent by nature. Yet the statewide proportion for which this factor was judged to be precipitating returns is only 5.6% of the total. Two of the regions, II and IV, show a proportion of 20.3% and 29.5% in this category. The other regions are much closer to the statewide proportion. The controlling finding is in Region VII (where the great bulk of study patients are), which, in quite the reverse, reported 1.6% of its total in this factor, as compared to the 5.6% statewide proportion. This accounts, in a large measure, for the overall low statewide proportion.

TABLE 26

AFTERCARE SERVICES WHICH COULD HAVE PREVENTED
PATIENTS' RETURN TO HOSPITAL IN REGION II

Aftercare	Number	Percentage	State Percentage
TOTAL	87	100.0%	100.0%
Regulation of medication	33	37.1	28.3
Counseling	12	13.7	14.5
Psychotherapy	11	12.6	13.1
Day treatment center	2	2.3	10.8
Alcoholics Anonymous	18	20.7	7.4
Sheltered living arrangements	3	3.2	7.4
Vocational rehabilitation	4	4.6	5.7
Resocialization	1	1.2	5.5
Other	—	—	—
No report	3	3.2	—

117

TABLE 27

AFTERCARE SERVICES WHICH COULD HAVE PREVENTED
PATIENTS' RETURN TO HOSPITAL IN REGION III

Aftercare	Number	Percentage	State Percentage
TOTAL	133	100.0%	100.0%
Regulation of medication	38	28.6	28.3
Counseling	21	15.7	14.5
Psychotherapy	20	15.0	13.1
Day treatment center	2	1.5	10.8
Alcoholics Anonymous	5	3.8	7.4
Sheltered living arrangements	31	23.3	7.4
Vocational rehabilitation	5	3.8	5.7
Resocialization	10	7.5	5.5
Other	9	6.7	5.7
No report	2	1.5	—

The following tables show the frequency distribution by regions with respect to the judgments of hospital staff as to aftercare services which could have been prevented patients' return.

The variations in Region II indicate that returned patients were judged to require much less day treatment center services (2.3%, as compared to 10.8%) than the reported statewide need, but considerably more services from Alcoholics Anonymous. Resocialization services were at a low level of need (1.2%, as compared to 5.5%) of the statewide proportion.

In Region III, there appears to be a substantial relative need, as shown in Table 27, for sheltered living arrangements for discharged patients, while the need for day treatment center services is low, as compared to the statewide picture.

TABLE 28
AFTERCARE SERVICES WHICH COULD HAVE PREVENTED
PATIENTS' RETURN TO HOSPITAL IN REGION IV

Aftercare	Number	Percentage	State Percentage
TOTAL	47	100.0%	100.0%
Regulation of medication	10	21.2	28.3
Counseling	10	21.2	14.5
Psychotherapy	7	14.8	13.1
Day treatment center	—	—	10.8
Alcoholics Anonymous	7	14.9	7.4
Sheltered living arrangements	4	8.5	7.4
Vocational rehabilitation	1	2.1	5.7
Resocialization	3	6.4	5.5
Other	5	10.6	5.7
No report	—	—	—

Region IV, again consistent with its experience, suggests twice the statewide need for Alcoholics Anonymous. In this region, the need for day treatment center services does not register on the scale at all.

In Region V, while consistent with the statewide proportions in most categories, a comparatively low need for sheltered living arrangements is registered.

Region VI shows little variance from the statewide picture. It falls below the day treatment center by more than half and is almost twice as frequent for resocialization services.

Region VII corresponds in most particulars to the statewide proportions. Day treatment centers are recorded at 14.9%, as against the 10.8% state percentage; and counseling services are below the state proportion.

It will be noted that in Region VIII there is an unusual distribution in the three principal services listed—

TABLE 29
AFTERCARE SERVICES WHICH COULD HAVE PREVENTED PATIENTS' RETURN TO HOSPITAL IN REGION V

Aftercare	Number	Percentage	State Percentage
TOTAL	136	100.0%	100.0%
Regulation of medication	53	39.0	28.3
Counseling	19	13.9	14.5
Psychotherapy	16	11.7	13.1
Day treatment center	17	12.5	10.8
Alcoholics Anonymous	5	3.6	7.4
Sheltered living arrangements	2	1.5	7.4
Vocational rehabilitation	8	5.8	5.7
Resocialization	7	5.2	5.5
Other	7	5.2	5.7
No report	2	1.5	—

TABLE 30
AFTERCARE SERVICES WHICH COULD HAVE PREVENTED PATIENTS' RETURN TO HOSPITAL IN REGION VI

Aftercare	Number	Percentage	State Percentage
TOTAL	98	100.0%	100.0%
Regulation of medication	27	27.5	28.3
Counseling	22	22.4	14.5
Psychotherapy	12	12.2	13.1
Day treatment centers	4	4.1	10.8
Alcoholics Anonymous	5	5.1	7.4
Sheltered living arrangements	8	8.2	7.4
Vocational rehabilitation	4	4.0	5.7
Resocialization	9	9.2	5.5
Other	7	7.1	5.7
No report	—	—	—

TABLE 31

AFTERCARE SERVICES WHICH COULD HAVE PREVENTED
PATIENTS' RETURN TO HOSPITAL IN REGION VII

Aftercare	Number	Percentage	State Percentage
TOTAL	1,053	100.0%	100.0%
Regulation of medication	310	29.4	28.3
Counseling	90	8.5	14.5
Psychotherapy	170	16.1	13.1
Day treatment centers	157	14.9	10.8
Alcoholics Anonymous	62	5.9	7.4
Sheltered living arrangements	67	6.3	7.4
Vocational rehabilitation	64	6.1	5.7
Resocialization	50	4.7	5.5
Other	68	6.5	5.7
No report	15	1.4	—

medication, counseling, and psychotherapy. In order to sustain community tenure, returned patients required, in the judgment of the hospital staff, less medication regulation, less psychotherapy, but much more counseling than the statewide proportions in these categories.

The frequency distribution of reasons aftercare services were not utilized by returned patients is shown in the following tables for each region.

In Region I, more than half of the returned patients refused aftercare services while out of hospital—56%, as compared to the 43.4% statewide proportion. However, in timely provision of services and planning for patients' use of them, the proportion is below the statewide percentage —14.5%, as compared to 24.9%.

The corrected figure (i.e., deducting the "Services not available" category from the total number) for Region I is 241.

In Region II, timeliness and effective planning of aftercare services do not constitute the problem represented in the statewide picture—13.8%, as compared to 24.9%. The corrected figure for **Region II** is 70.

TABLE 32
AFTERCARE SERVICES WHICH COULD HAVE PREVENTED PATIENTS' RETURN TO HOSPITAL IN REGION VIII

Aftercare	Number	Percentage	State Percentage
TOTAL	202	100.0%	100.0%
Regulation of medication	40	19.8	28.3
Counseling	75	37.1	14.5
Psychotherapy	9	4.4	13.1
Day treatment centers	16	7.9	10.8
Alcoholics Anonymous	18	8.9	7.4
Sheltered living arrangements	17	8.4	7.4
Vocational rehabilitation	12	5.9	5.7
Resocialization	5	2.5	5.5
Other	4	2.0	5.7
No report	6	2.9	—

TABLE 33
REASONS AFTERCARE SERVICES WERE NOT UTILIZED BY RETURNED PATIENTS IN REGION I

Reasons	Number	Percentage	State Percentage
TOTAL	312	100.0%	100.0%
Patient refused service	175	56.0	43.4
Service not available	71	22.7	20.1
Service not provided soon enough or irregularly	27	8.7	15.7
Ineffectual planning	18	5.8	9.2
Other	11	3.5	5.4
No report	10	3.2	6.1

TABLE 34

REASONS AFTERCARE SERVICES WERE NOT UTILIZED
BY RETURNED PATIENTS IN REGION II

Reasons	Number	Percentage	State Percentage
TOTAL	87	100.0%	100.0%
Patient refused service	43	49.4	43.4
Service not available	17	19.5	20.1
Service not provided soon enough or irregularly	7	8.0	15.7
Ineffectual planning	5	5.8	9.2
Other	5	5.8	5.4
No report	10	11.4	6.1

TABLE 35

REASONS AFTERCARE SERVICES WERE NOT UTILIZED
BY RETURNED PATIENTS IN REGION III

Reasons	Number	Percentage	State Percentage
TOTAL	146	100.0%	100.0%
Patient refused service	57	39.1	43.4
Service not available	24	11.6	20.1
Service not provided soon enough or irregularly	27	16.8	15.7
Ineffectual planning	13	8.9	9.2
Other	14	10.0	5.4
No report	11	7.5	6.1

In Region III, the proportion appears to correspond fairly closely to the statewide proportion.

The corrected figure for Region III is 122.

Region IV shows the highest percentage of patients who refused services—76.6%, as compared to the 43.4%

statewide. The nonavailability problem is inconsequential —4.2%, as compared to the statewide proportion of 20.1%.

The corrected figure for Region IV is 45.

In Region V, the "service not available" factor is 11.8%, as compared to the 20.1% statewide. A higher

TABLE 36

REASONS AFTERCARE SERVICES WERE NOT UTILIZED
BY RETURNED PATIENTS IN REGION IV

Reasons	Number	Percentage	State Percentage
TOTAL	47	100.0%	100.0%
Patient refused service	36	76.6	43.4
Service not available	2	4.2	20.1
Service not provided soon enough or irregularly	—	—	15.7
Ineffectual planning	4	8.5	9.2
Other	1	2.2	5.4
No report	4	8.5	6.1

TABLE 37

REASONS AFTERCARE SERVICES WERE NOT UTILIZED
BY RETURNED PATIENTS IN REGION V

Reasons	Number	Percentage	State Percentage
TOTAL	136	100.0%	100.0%
Patient refused service	70	51.5	43.4
Service not available	16	11.8	20.1
Service not provided soon enough or irregularly	31	22.8	15.7
Ineffectual planning	8	5.8	9.2
Other	9	6.6	5.4
No report	2	1.8	6.1

percentage—51.5%—refused service than the statewide proportion of 43.4%.

The corrected figure for Region V is 120.

Region VI shows a pattern which corresponds to the statewide picture.

The corrected figure for Region VI is 78.

TABLE 38

REASONS AFTERCARE SERVICES WERE NOT UTILIZED
BY RETURNED PATIENTS IN REGION VI

Reasons	Number	Percentage	State Percentage
TOTAL	97	100.0%	100.0%
Patient refused service	40	41.2	43.4
Service not available	19	19.6	20.1
Service not provided soon enough or irregularly	17	19.5	15.7
Ineffectual planning	11	11.5	9.2
Other	8	8.2	5.4
No report	2	2.0	6.1

TABLE 39

REASONS AFTERCARE SERVICES WERE NOT UTILIZED
BY RETURNED PATIENTS IN REGION VII

Reasons	Number	Percentage	State Percentage
TOTAL	1,054	100.0%	100.0%
Patient refused service	410	38.9	43.4
Service not available	238	22.5	20.1
Service not provided soon enough or irregularly	176	16.7	15.7
Ineffectual planning	103	9.8	9.2
Other	51	4.8	5.4
No report	76	7.2	6.1

TABLE 40
REASONS AFTERCARE SERVICES WERE NOT UTILIZED
BY RETURNED PATIENTS IN REGION VIII

Reasons	Number	Percentage	State Percentage
TOTAL	201	100.0%	100.0%
Patient refused service	73	36.3	43.4
Service not available	32	15.9	20.1
Service not provided soon enough or irregularly	41	20.4	15.7
Ineffectual planning	29	14.4	9.2
Other	13	6.4	5.4
No report	13	6.4	6.1

Region VII, which dominates all others numerically, reflects the statewide picture, just as it influences it. The "patient refused service" is lower (38.9%) than the state percentage of 43.4%.

The corrected figure for Region VII is 816.

Ineffectual planning and lack of timeliness in provision of aftercare services are recorded in Region VIII at 34.8%, as compared to the statewide 24.9%. Fewer patients refused aftercare services than the statewide proportion—36.3%, as compared to 43.4%.

The corrected figure for Region VIII is 169.

In summary, it can be seen that there is a wide range in the nonutilization rate by regions. The range is from 83.9% in Region V to 29.4% in Region IV. This variation makes it possible to set up an appropriate test of the relationship of return rates and utilization rates. The actual test was done (see Chapter 4), revealing a correlation between these two variables in five of the eight regions, leading to the conclusion that the higher the rate of utilization of aftercare services by ex-patients, the lower the rate of return to hospital.

APPENDICES:

APPENDIX
I

RESEARCH QUESTIONS AND HYPOTHESES

Most studies proceed on the basis of implicit or explicit assumptions and questions with some tentative answers. The framework and focus for this study and analysis were provided by certain assumptions developed in the Task Force Report on Aftercare. For purposes of this study, these were formulated into hypotheses providing tentative answers to the following specific research questions. (Rules for testing hypotheses were spelled out in advance).

RESEARCH QUESTIONS AND HYPOTHESES

1. In a one-year period, what proportion of patients leaving the eighteen state mental hospitals in Pennsylvania are judged by the hospital staff to require aftercare services in the eight regions?

The Task Force hypothesizes that 85% of all patients leaving state hospitals will require one or more aftercare services.

2. What is the frequency distribution of specific aftercare services recommended at discharge in the eight regions?

The Task Force Report hypothesizes that reemployment and resocialization services constitute the principal aftercare needs of patients at discharge.

3. To what extent are recommended aftercare services available in the eight regions to patients who leave hospital?

The Task Force hypothesizes that: (a) aftercare facilities are insufficient in number throughout the state; (b) they are primarily available in the large metropolitan areas of the state.

4. What proportion of patients return to hospital from the eight regions within one year after leaving hospital?

The Task Force hypothesizes that the state return percentage will approximate the national return percentage of between 35% and 38%.

5. What are the most frequent reasons given for readmission to hospital?

The Task Force hypothesizes that the most frequent cause of patients' return to hospital within one year after leaving is the lack of aftercare services.

6. What proportion of ex-patients utilize available recommended aftercare services in the eight regions?

The Task Force hypothesizes that a major problem in the aftercare program is low patient utilization of available recommended aftercare services.

7. What is the relationship between the rate of return and utilization of available recommended aftercare services in the eight regions?

The Task Force hypothesizes that the higher the rate of utilization of available aftercare services, the lower the rate of return.

8. What other factors appear to be related to rate of return to hospital?

RULES FOR TESTING HYPOTHESES

The Task Force Report hypotheses were tested for possible acceptance or rejection by the results of the Aftercare Study. If any of the hypotheses were rejected, specific changes were indicated for the proposals and recommendations of the Task Force on Aftercare of the Comprehensive Mental Health Plan (see Chapter 5).

The results of the aftercare study were also used to derive additional hypotheses about the defined research problems and to indicate possible additional problems for further research.

The rules for accepting or rejecting the Task Force hypotheses were as follows:

1. Eighty-five percent of all patients leaving state hospitals will require one or more aftercare services.

Rule: If less than (85% — *e*), reject; if (85% — *e*) or over, accept, where *(e)* is an "allowable error" of 10%.

2. Reemployment and resocialization services constitute the principal aftercare needs of ex-patients.

Rule: If the combined recommendations for these services exceed the number of recommendations of all other aftercare services, accept; if not, reject.

3. (a) Aftercare facilities are insufficient in number throughout the state. . . .

Rule: If less than 75% of all recommended aftercare services are available in each of the regions, accept; above 75%, reject.

(b) They are available primarily in the large metropolitan areas of the state.*

Rule: If Region I and Region VII each have the highest percentage of available aftercare services, exceeding five of the eight regions by 50% or more, accept; if below 50%, reject.

4. The state return percentage will approximate the national return percentage of between 35% and 38%.

Rule: If the return percentage is between 35% and 38%, accept; if not, reject.

5. The most frequent cause of patients' return to hospital within one year of leaving is the lack of aftercare services.

Rule: If the frequency is highest for lack of aftercare services, accept; if not, reject.

6. A major problem in the aftercare program is low utilization of available services.

Rule: If percentage is 50% or less, accept; more than 50%, reject.

7. The higher the utilization of available aftercare services, the lower the returns to hospital.

Rule: If the rank order of utilization rate by regions corresponds to the return rate in five of the eight regions, accept; if not, reject.

8. Other factors related to rate of return. No hypothesis to be tested; derivations to be obtained from study data.

*Region I includes Pittsburgh; Region VII includes Philadelphia.

APPENDIX
II

Definitions of terms and instructions are given below for those items on the forms that are not self-explanatory. If the information for any item on the forms is unknown, please enter the letters "NK".

Record of Patient Leaving the Hospital (MH 511)

Item 4. *Type of removal*—Check the proper item to indicate whether patient left the hospital on trial visit or family care or was discharged (removed from the books).

> *Trial visit*—Include patients on leave for possible adjustment to community life. Include those in their own home, CID institutions and nursing homes. Do not include patients in family care as defined below.

> *Family care*—Include patients placed in the community in private families other than their own, under the supervision of the hospital.

Item 5. *Sex*—Enter "M" for male, "F" for female.

Item 9. *Occupation*—Under major occupation, enter the occupation or profession which the patient pursued the longest part of his working life. It is the one out of several the patient may have had that accounted for the greatest number of years of his working life. If the patient was retired prior to hospitalization, enter his usual occupation, followed by the entry "ret."

132

RECORD OF PATIENT LEAVING THE HOSPITAL
Pennsylvania State Mental Hospitals

1. Hospital_____ 2. Name _____ 3. Case no. _____

4. Type of removal (check):   Trial visit_____ Family care_____ Direct discharge_____

7. County where patient

5. Sex_____   6. Race (check): White____Nonwhite_____   will reside_____

8. Marital status (check):
   Married_____ Widowed_____ Divorced_____ Separated_____ Never married_____

9. Occupations: Major _____ Secondary _____

10. Mental   11. Number of   12. Date of current
    Disorder(code):_____   previous admissions_____   admission _____

13. Number of removals   14. Date of current   15. Age on current
    since Oct. 1, 1962_____   removal _____   removal _____

16. Type of   17. Living arrangements after leaving hospital (check):
    commitment (check):   Alone.................... _____   Nursing home or county home _____
    Voluntary................. _____   With spouse .... _____   Foster home or family care... _____
    Med. Cert. Standard.... _____   With other relative(s)_____   Other........................ .... _____
    Med. Cert. Emergency _____   With nonrelative(s)... _____   Unknown........................... _____
    Judicial Procedure ..... _____

18. Treatment one year prior to current release (check applicable items):
    Psychotropic drugs_____ Psychotherapy: Individual_____ Group_____
    Electroshock _____ Other (specify) _____

19. Medication(s) prescribed on leaving hospital (check applicable items):
    Tranquilizer_____ Energizer_____ Other_____ None_____

20. Prescribed medication(s) to be provided by (check):
    Patient and/or family..... _____   Public Assistance_____
    Hospital...................... _____   Other (specify) _____

21. Was a pre-leave plan arranged? (check): Yes____ No____

22.	Services needed Col. 1 (check)	Are needed services available? Col. 2 "yes" or "no"	Who will provided services for patient? Col. 3 (complete)
a. Regulation of medication			
b. Psychotherapy			
c. Counseling			
d. Vocational rehabilitation			
e. Sheltered living arrangement			
f. Day treatment center			
g. Resocialization experience			
h. Alcoholics Anonymous			
i. V.N.A. or Public Health Nurse			
j. Public Assistance			
k. Other (specify)_____			
l. None			

23. Prognosis for patient's adjustment outside the hospital (check):
    Good_____ Fair_____ Guarded_____

24. Is patient immediately, or with some additional training, likely able to work at gainful employment? (check):
    Yes_____ No_____
    If yes, complete questions 25 thru 34 on reverse side.
    If no, state reason _____

MH 511 - 10-62 (50)

25. Highest grade of school __completed__ (in years)_____

26. Length of time patient was employable, during his lifetime_____ Years_____ Months

27. Number of different jobs (of at least 6 months duration) patient held in the last 10 years _____

28. Longest period of employment on one job, during his lifetime_____Years_____ Months

29. Condition under which patient __usually__ left job (check one):
    Patient left job
    To accept another position.....................____
    Quit with no future employment plans......____
    Because of mental illness..................... ____
    Other (specify)_____
    Discharged................................ ____

30. Major type of work assignment in hospital (check one):
    Service..................... ____
    Agricultural.............. ____
    Industrial
       Unskilled................ ____
       Semi-skilled............ ____
    Clerical..................... ____
    Other....................... ____
    None....................... ____

31. Supervision required in hospital work assignment (check): Close_____ Minimal_____

32. Work performance in hospital work assignment (check): Poor_____ Fair_____ Good_____

33. Job readiness on leaving hospital (check): Poor_____ Fair_____ Good_____

34. Is patient returning to former position? (check): Yes_____ No _____

    Vague titles such as simply "laborer" or the name of the company for which the patient worked should be avoided. Sufficiently descriptive titles of occupations or professions are: carpenter; plumber; lawyer; dentist; grade school teacher; department store salesman; railroad laborer; foreman in aircraft factory; housewife; etc. If the patient was in school at the time of admission, enter "high school student," "grade school student," etc. If the patient was not in school or had no occupation or profession as defined above, enter "None."

    Under secondary occupation, enter the occupation or profession which the patient pursued for the next to longest part of his working life. Follow instructions as for major occupation above. If patient had no secondary occupation, enter "None."

Item 10. *Mental disorder*—Enter the APA numerical diagnostic code.

Item 11. *Number of previous admissions*—Enter the number of previous admissions (exclude current admission) to any *inpatient* psychiatric facility. Include admissions to a state hospital (in Pennsylvania or another state), psychiatric ward of a general hospital, private mental hospital, VA hospital.

134

Item 13. *Number of removals since October 1, 1962*—Enter the number of times since October 1, 1962 the patient has left the hospital on trial visit, family care, or direct discharge. The first time he leaves, enter "1"; should he return and again leave the hospital, enter "2", etc. Removals for temporary visit, other authorized absence, or unauthorized absence are *not* included as "removals" in this item.

Item 15. *Age on removal*—Enter the age (in years) as of last birthday at time of removal from the hospital. If unknown, enter the approximate age.

Item 16. *Type of commitment*—Check the appropriate item to indicate the initial type of commitment involved when the patient entered the hospital for his current admission.

Item 21. *Was a preleave plan arranged?*—A preleave plan is defined as a *minimum* of one interview with the *patient* relative to planning for living arrangements, medication, services needed, etc.

Item 22. *Services needed* (Col. 1)—Check the service(s) (maximum of 4) which are felt the patient needs to help him make a successful adjustment to community life.

Are needed services available? (Col. 2)—Enter "yes" or "no" only for those services that were checked as needed in column 1. Enter "yes" if service will be available to the patient after he leaves the hospital. Enter "no" if the service is not available or if the service is available but inadequate.

Who will provide services for patient? (Col. 3)—For each item checked in column 1, enter in column 3 the position of the individual or the type of organization or institution that will provide these services. Examples follow.

   a. *Regulation of medication*—Can be under the supervision of the state hospital, outpatient clinic, community clinic, private physician.
   b. *Psychotherapy*—Defined as treatment by purely psychological means given by a dynamically oriented person.
   c. *Counseling*—Can be provided by state hospital staff, hospital or community clinic, social agency, clergyman, etc.
   g. *Resocialization experience*—Defined as any type of social activity that assists the patient in developing interests, participate in group activity, and improves his interpersonal relationships. Include such activities as attending church, joining clubs, taking dance lessons, etc.

135

Item 24. *Is patient immediately or with some additional training likely able to work at gainful employment?* Examples of reasons patients will not be able to work at gainful employment after leaving the hospital are: age (the very young or aged), physical disability, household duties, inability to adjust to employment situation.

Item 26. *Length of time patient was employable before entering hospital*—Include in this item the length of time patient was employable whether employed or unemployed.

Item 30. *Major type of work assignment in hospital*

Service—Include domestic, dietary, laundry, ward aides, etc. assignments.

Agricultural—Include work on the farm, truck garden, dairy, grounds crew.

Industrial—Include general labor crews, tradesmen helpers, etc.

Item 32. *Work performance in hospital work assignment*—In rating patient's work performance consider quality and quantity of work, acceptance of instructions, relationship with supervisor and co-workers, work habits and attitudes.

Item 33. *Job readiness on leaving hospital*—In evaluating patient's job readiness consider his motivation for work, abilities, salable job skills, self-confidence as a worker, dependability, initiative.

RECORD OF PATIENT RETURNING TO HOSPITAL (MH 512)

Items 4 and 5. Should agree with items 4 and 14 on Record of Patient Leaving the Hospital.

Item 7. *Services which could have prevented patient's return to hospital*—For those services (maximum of 4) that if provided could have prevented the patient's return to the hospital, enter the code number that represents the reason the service was not provided.

Item 11. *Was patient employable while out of the hospital?*— Examples of reasons patients were not employable while out of the hospital are: age (the very young or aged), physical disability, household duties.

Item 14. *Jobs held*—Enter the type of jobs held, not the name of employer. Examples: truck driver, farmer, retail salesman, waitress.

136

RECORD OF PATIENT RETURNING TO HOSPITAL
Pennsylvania State Mental Hospitals

1. Hospital_____ 2. Name _____ 3. Case no _____

4. Type of removal (check): Trial visit_____ Family care_____ Direct discharge_____
   If patient has a different case no. from the one when removed, enter previous case no._____ .

5. Date of current   6. Date of current
   removal_____   return to hospital _____

7. Services which could have prevented patient's return to hospital (code applicable items):
   Regulation of medication.......................... _____   Day treatment center............................... _____
   Psychotherapy....................................... _____   Resocialization experience..................... _____
   Counseling... _____   Alcoholics Anonymous........................... _____
   Vocational rehabilitation......................... _____   V.N.A. or Public Health Nurse................ _____
   Sheltered living arrangement................... _____   Public Assistance................................ _____
              Other (specify)_____

         Codes for reasons service was not provided
              1 - Service not available
              2 - Patient refused service
              3 - Service should have been provided sooner and/or more regularly
              4 - Patient moved from area
              5 - Ineffectual planning
              6 - Other

   If you feel no service could have prevented the patient's return to the hospital, check here_____

8. What primarily precipitated the patient's return to the hospital? (check one):
   Premature release.................................... _____   Inability to cope with stressful situations...... _____
   Release against medical advice................. _____   Excessive drinking................................... _____
   Refused or discontinued medication............ _____   Different symptoms from previous illness....... _____
   Negative family environment..................... _____   Other (specify) _____
   Other environmental problems................... _____   Unknown.. _____

9. If patient refused or discontinued medication, give primary reason (check one):
   Cost of drug... _____   Other (specify) _____ ___
   Distance too far to obtain drug................. _____   Unknown.. _____
   Patient suffered side effects................... _____
   Time elapsed between discontinuance of medication and patient's return to the hospital_____ months

10. Was there any change in living arrangements since patient left hospital? (check):
    Yes_____ No _____ Unknown _____

11. Was patient employable while out of the hospital? (check): Yes_____ No_____
    If yes, complete questions 12 thru 15.
    If no, state reason _____

12. Did patient actively seek employment while out of hospital? (check): Yes_____ No _____

13. Number of jobs (of any duration) held while out of hospital_____

14.   Jobs held (3 months or longer)   Length of time employed
    a._____   a._____
    b._____   b._____
    c._____   c._____

15. Condition under which patient usually left above jobs (check one):
    Patient left job
       To accept another position.................................. _____
       Quit with no future employment plans................... _____
       Because of mental illness.................................. _____
       Other (specify)_____ _____
    Discharged... _____

                                                         MH 512 - 10-62 (50)

APPENDIX
III

(4) Aftercare and rehabilitation will be effected through the development and expansion of a range of community-based facilities including sheltered workshops, halfway houses, retraining programs, homemaking services, and foster home care. There will be sought a reworking of employment and compensation laws insofar as these now constitute a handicap to rehabilitation. (p. 16)

An Integrated Summary of Task Force Recommendations

1. *Comprehensive Mental Health Program*

   a) Definition of Comprehensive Mental Health Program

   (1) A comprehensive mental health program should be a continuum of integrated and coordinated mental health services emphasizing flexibility and continuity and made available to the community according to need. These services should comprise an optimal blending of prevention and detection with diagnosis, treatment and rehabilitation and should be supported by ongoing research and program evaluation.

*From Commonwealth of Pennsylvania. "The Comprehensive Mental Health Plan," C. J. Bodarky, Ed. (Health and Welfare Building, Harrisburg, Pa.), 1965. Page numbers in parentheses refer to this publication.

b) Principles of Operation of the Comprehensive
Mental Health Program

(1) There should be as little disruption as possible of the relationships of a person with family, school and neighborhood, unless of course, such disruption is a desired circumstance of treatment.

(2) A specific person or agency should be designated as responsible for steering and coordinating the services for the individual patient or client. The optimal application of this principle demands high levels of communication and cooperation among services.

(3) To enhance appropriate referrals, the evaluation process should discriminate between therapeutic services and those broad-based care services which provide support.

(4) Without damaging the principle of confidentiality, care and treatment services should be pursued on the "open" principle, i.e., information about the individual problem be readily transmitted between treating agencies, that transfer of cases be unimpeded and service unbroken and unduplicated. This is of special significance in view of the community mental health center's mandated procedure for coordinated services.

(5) The delivery of these services should occur as close to the people who utilize such services as possible. Delivery systems should be developed and administered at the community level and probably on a county basis, given the fact that counties are the most logical government unit to assume mental health responsibilities at the community level. (p. 33)

(4) Aftercare and Rehabilitation

Aftercare and rehabilitation services are intended to maintain the continuity of treatment. These services include a wide range of facilities: sheltered workshops, rehabilitation centers, halfway houses.

a. There should be comprehensive care in nursing homes.

b. Rehabilitation and aftercare services should be encouraged and subsidized.

c. Any plan for a rehabilitation and aftercare service program should provide for local direction and administration of the program.

d. Payments to nursing homes should be increased to a more realistic figure so that services can be improved accordingly.

e. Low cost, good quality nursing homes should be encouraged and subsidized.

f. The funding of the rehabilitation and aftercare program should be patterned on a multiple-source support aim, using tax funds and private funds to guarantee adequate financial support for the program. A system of financial support should be developed, particularly as it refers to private organizations and agencies which are called upon to provide rehabilitation and aftercare services.

g. Rehabilitation and aftercare services should be community based as close as possible to the patients' home environment.

h. There should be establishment of those community supports which would enable the older person to continue to remain in the community as long as he is physically or mentally able to do so. Among these should be included:

(1) homemaker services

(2) home medical care programs

(3) day care centers

(4) Other rehabilitation services such as sheltered workshops and part-time employment opportunities (p. 48 & 49)

(15) High priority should be given to the development of a plan for training, recruitment, and development of specialized staff to perform three types of operating functions in rehabilitation and aftercare.

a. Community organization specialist

b. Counselor or caseworker

c. Rehabilitation worker.

Two training centers should be established, one in Western Pennsylvania and one in Eastern Pennsylvania, each connected with the graduate departments of a major university. (p. 59)

(7) Medical

Approximately 60% of the patients who leave state hospitals are placed on psychotropic drugs. Surveys indicate that half of these patients receive supervision of their medication from the hospital and that the remainder obtain supervision of medication from their private physician. Current research also indicates that public health nurses can assist patients to accommodate successfully to home care programs.

140

(8) Social Services

It is estimated that 85% of patients who leave mental hospitals and/or their families require counseling and other assistance from social service agencies. As noted above, these services should be available in precare services to prevent hospitalization.

(9) Vocational Rehabilitation

Rehabilitation services cover the areas of vocation rehabilitation, sheltered workshops and halfway houses or residential settings in the community. The Pennsylvania Bureau of Vocational Rehabilitation now serves 15% of the 12,000 discharged patients from our state mental institutions. It is estimated that as much as 40% of all discharged patients (25,000 patients per year) are in need of this service.

(11) Sheltered Workshops

Sheltered workshops for patients leaving mental institutions are often required to evaluate the employability of an individual, estimate his ego strength, prepare him for work, teach him basic job skills or, where required, to afford him a semipermanent occupational haven. Because former patients often have very low level of motivation toward work, it has been difficult at this time to adequately assess the need for this service. (p. 69 & 70)

Recommendations for Precare and Aftercare

(1) Every Mental Health Center should develop an extensive program for precare and aftercare, whether all of the services are provided in one building, or in a cluster of agencies.

(2) Every catchment area should have a "Services Coordinator" responsible for knowledge of services available in the area, and for bringing together the patient and the services. For the present planning period one coordinator is suggested for each catchment area.

(3) The Office of Mental Health should set up guidelines and suggestions which will assist the Services Coordinator to formulate programs for the catchment area.

Recommendations for Rehabilitation

There is a considerable overlap between aftercare and rehabilitation; however, social rehabilitation and vocational rehabilitation are usually thought of as an additional type of aftercare, and it is these services which are being considered here.

141

(1) Early attention should be given to establishing halfway houses, foster homes, or other types of residential facilities for discharged or "on leave" patients.

(2) Consideration should be given to organizing social clubs for former patients in those catchment areas where no such clubs exist. It is suggested that local citizen groups, such as Mental Health Associations, be asked to sponsor these clubs.

(3) A network of sheltered workshops and employment centers, and a regional vocational training center should be established.

(4) One vocational rehabilitation counselor should be assigned to each catchment area.

(5) A better understanding of what "recovery" means should be achieved with employers through a strong public educational program conducted by the Mental Health Center, working closely with a state-employed regional educator, and with existing civic agencies. (p. 89)

APPENDIX
IV

STATE MENTAL HOSPITAL PERSONNEL

The following charts indicate the 1964 treatment staff complements by classifications, as compared to American Psychiatric Association standards:

REGION I

Dixmont State Hospital

	Current Staff Complement	APA Standard for Staff Complement	Deficit in Staff Complement by APA Standard
Physicians	4	12	8
Psychologists	6	6	6
Nurses	24	46	22
Social workers	4	9	5
Attendants	162	180	18
Other "activities" personnel	17	17	—
TOTALS:	217	270	59

Psychiatric Aftercare

Mayview State Hospital

	Current Staff Complement	APA Standard for Staff Complement	Deficit in Staff Complement by APA Standard
Physicians	40	47	7
Psychologists	7	14	7
Nurses	82	245	163
Social workers	12	38	26
Attendants	572	640	68
Other "activities" personnel	75	75	—
TOTALS:	788	1,059	271

Torrance State Hospital

	Current Staff Complement	APA Standard for Staff Complement	Deficit in Staff Complement by APA Standard
Physicians	10	34	24
Psychologists	4	9	5
Nurses	44	209	165
Social workers	9	33	24
Attendants	537	624	87
Other "activities" personnel	70	70	—
TOTALS:	674	979	305

Woodville State Hospital

	Current Staff Complement	APA Standard for Staff Complement	Deficit in Staff Complement by APA Standard
Physicians	27	46	19
Psychologists	7	9	2
Nurses	57	238	181
Social workers	9	23	14
Attendants	413	550	137
Other "activities" personnel	61	61	—
TOTALS:	574	927	353

REGION II

Warren State Hospital

	Current Staff Complement	APA Standard for Staff Complement	Deficit in Staff Complement by APA Standard
Physicians	40	40	0
Psychologists	1	8	7
Nurses	66	213	147
Social workers	8	50	42
Attendants	402	580	78
Other "activities" personnel	117	117	—
TOTALS:	634	1,008	274

REGION III

Hollidaysburg State Hospital

	Current Staff Complement	APA Standard for Staff Complement	Deficit in Staff Complement by APA Standard
Physicians	14	16	2
Psychologists	2	4	2
Nurses	35	52	17
Social workers	5	20	15
Attendants	146	182	32
Other "activities" personnel	10	10	—
TOTALS:	212	284	68

Somerset State Hospital

	Current Staff Complement	APA Standard for Staff Complement	Deficit in Staff Complement by APA Standard
Physicians	4	18	14
Psychologists	1	6	5
Nurses	25	61	36
Social workers	4	9	5
Attendants	159	159	—
Other "activities" personnel	17	17	—
TOTALS:	210	270	60

REGION IV

Danville State Hospital

	Current Staff Complement	APA Standard for Staff Complement	Deficit in Staff Complement by APA Standard
Physicians	23	52	29
Psychologists	5	8	3
Nurses	124	163	39
Social workers	9	32	23
Attendants	427	474	47
Other "activities" personnel	54	54	—
TOTALS:	642	783	141

REGION V

Clarks Summit State Hospital

	Current Staff Complement	APA Standard for Staff Complement	Deficit in Staff Complement by APA Standard
Physicians	12	15	3
Psychologists	2	2	—
Nurses	56	85	29
Social workers	9	14	5
Attendants	169	244	75
Other "activities" personnel	28	28	—
TOTALS:	276	388	112

Retreat State Hospital

At the time of the study, the hospital was going through a complete reorganization, with transfer of patients and staff, so that comparable data on staff complements were not available.

146

REGION VI

Allentown State Hospital

	Current Staff Complement	APA Standard for Staff Complement	Deficit in Staff Complement by APA Standard
Physicians	24	33	9
Psychologists	4	11	7
Nurses	73	96	23
Social workers	14	42	28
Attendants	333	424	91
Other "activities" personnel	28	28	—
TOTALS	476	634	158

Wernersville State Hospital

	Current Staff Complement	APA Standard for Staff Complement	Deficit in Staff Complement by APA Standard
Physicians	16	27	11
Psychologists	6	6	0
Nurses	56	133	77
Social workers	8	21	13
Attendants	266	364	98
Other "activities" personnel	48	48	—
TOTALS:	400	599	199

REGION VII

Philadelphia State Hospital

	Current Staff Complement	APA Standard for Staff Complement	Deficit in Staff Complement by APA Standard
Physicians	64	90	26
Psychologists	14	21	7
Nurses	102	443	341
Social workers	22	100	78
Attendants	882	1,260	378
Other "activities" personnel	61	61	—
TOTALS:	1,145	1,975	830

147

Psychiatric Aftercare

Norristown State Hospital

	Current Staff Complement	APA Standard for Staff Complement	Deficit in Staff Complement by APA Standard
Physicians	50	50	0
Psychologists	11	11	0
Nurses	93	200	107
Social workers	21	42	21
Attendants	638	765	127
Other "activities" personnel	49	49	—
TOTALS:	862	1,117	255

Haverford State Hospital

	Current Staff Complement	APA Standard for Staff Complement	Deficit in Staff Complement by APA Standard
Physicians	15	15	0
Psychologists	6	6	0
Nurses	49	57	8
Social workers	16	31	15
Attendants	274	274	—
Other "activities" personnel	28	28	—
TOTALS:	388	411	23

Embreeville State Hospital

	Current Staff Complement	APA Standard for Staff Complement	Deficit in Staff Complement by APA Standard
Physicians	21	21	0
Psychologists	7	7	0
Nurses	40	85	45
Social workers	8	24	16
Attendants	283	283	—
Other "activities" personnel	56	56	—
TOTALS:	415	476	61

REGION VIII

Harrisburg State Hospital

	Current Staff Complement	APA Standard for Staff Complement	Deficit in Staff Complement by APA Standard
Physicians	18	27	9
Psychologists	5	5	0
Nurses	48	144	96
Social workers	11	40	29
Attendants	482	487	5
Other "activities" personnel	52	52	—
TOTALS:	616	755	139

Bibliography

Books

Albee, G. W. *Mental Health Manpower Trends.* (New York: Basic Books, Monograph Series No. 3) 1959.

Arieti, S. (Ed.) *American Handbook of Psychiatry.* 2 vols., (New York: Basic Books) 1959, Vol. II, p. 1877.

Crutcher, H. B. *Foster Home Care for Mental Patients.* (New York: Commonwealth Fund) 1944.

DeWitt, Henrietta. *Foster Care Placement of State Mental Hospital Patients: Maryland Plan, 1954.* (Maryland State Department of Mental Hygiene, Baltimore, Md.).

Fein, R. *Economics of Mental Illness.* (New York: Basic Books, Monograph Series No. 2) 1958.

Felix, R. H., *et al. Mental Health and Social Welfare.* (New York: Columbia University Press) 1961.

Freeman, H. E. and Simmons, O. G. *The Mental Patient Comes Home.* (New York: John Wiley and Sons) 1963.

Hollingshead, A. B. and Redlich, F. C. *Social Class and Mental Illness.* (New York: John Wiley and Sons) 1958.

Joint Commission on Mental Illness and Health. *Action for Mental Health.* (New York: Basic Books) 1961.

National Association of Social Workers. *Social Work Yearbook.* R. H. Kurtz, Ed. New York, 1960, pp. 451-458.

Srole, L., Langer T. S., Michael, S. T., Opler, M. K., and Rennie, T.A.C. *Mental Health in the Metropolis: The Midtown Manhattan Study.* Vol. I (New York: McGraw-Hill) 1962.

Articles

Albee, G. W. "The Manpower Crisis in Mental Health," *American Journal of Public Health.* December 1960, Vol. 50, No. 12.

151

Bierer, J. "Great Britain's Therapeutic Social Clubs," *Mental Hospitals, The Journal of Hospital and Community Psychiatry.* April 1962, Vol. 13, p. 203, (American Psychiatric Association, Washington, D.C.).

Bravos, T. A., Bay, A. P., and Fox, W. "Aftercare, Intermediate Care and Rehabilitation," *Mental Hospitals, The Journal of Hospital and Community Psychiatry,* February 1962, Vol. 13, pp. 104-106.

Conte, W. R., Rew, W. B., Wolfrom, E. "Aftercare Program for Discharged Mental Patients," *Northwest Medicine,* May 1963, Vol. 62, p. 341.

Cumming, E. "Allocation of Care to the Mentally Ill, American Style," *Organizing for Community Welfare,* H. N. Zold, Ed., (Chicago: Quadrangle Books) 1967.

Cumming, E. and Cumming, J. "Some Questions on Community Care," *Canada's Mental Health,* November-December 1965, Vol. XIII, No. 6, (Mental Health Division, Department of National Health and Welfare, Ottawa, Canada).

Felix, R. H. "Breakthrough in Mental Illness," *Health, Education and Welfare Indicators,* November 1963, pp. XXXV-XXXVI.

Forrest, F. M., Geiter, C. W., Snow, H. L., and Steinbach, M. "Drug Maintenance Problems of Rehabilitated Mental Patients," *American Journal of Psychiatry,* July 1964, Vol. 121, No. 1, p. 33.

Free, S. M. and Dodd, D. F. "Aftercare for Discharged Mental Patients: Report of a Conference on a Five-State Study," *Mental Health in Virginia,* Vol. 12, No. 11, Summer 1961. (Department of Mental Hygiene and Hospitals, Richmond, Va.).

Fromm-Reichmann, F., Selected Papers of, D. M. Bullard, Ed. *Psychoanalysis and Psychotherapy,* (Chicago: University of Chicago Press) 1959.

Funkhouser, J. B. "Mental Hygiene Clinic Activity in Aftercare," *Mental Health in Virginia,* Summer 1962, Vol. 12, No. 14, (Department of Mental Hygiene and Hospitals, Richmond, Va.).

Hoffman, H. J. "Paid Employment As a Rehabilitative Technique in a State Mental Hospital: A Demonstration," *Mental*

Hygiene, April 1965, Vol. 49, No. 2, p. 193, (National Association for Mental Health, Inc., New York).

Horwitz, J. J. "Social Work Skills in the Rehabilitation of Mental Patients," *Psychiatric Quarterly Supplement, Canada's Mental Health.* February 1963. (Department of National Health and Welfare, Ottawa, Canada).

Huseth, B. "England's Halfway Houses," *Mental Hospitals, The Journal of Hospital and Community Psychiatry.* August 1962, Vol. 13, p. 422. (American Psychiatric Association, Washington, D.C.).

Jaquith, W. L. "A Mail-Order Drug Program for Discharged Patients," *Mental Hospitals. The Journal of Hospital and Community Psychiatry,* November 1961, Vol. 12, p. 34. (American Psychiatric Association, Washington, D.C.).

Kantor, D. and Greenblatt, M. "Wellmet: Halfway to Community Rehabilitation," *Mental Hospitals. The Journal of Hospital and Community Psychiatry,* March 1962, Vol. 13, p. 146. (American Psychiatric Association, Washington, D.C.).

Kubelli, G. E., Levis, J., and Havens, L. L. "Hospital-Based Vocational Rehabilitation Programs," *Mental Hygiene.* October 1965, Vol. 49, No. 4, p. 501. (National Association for Mental Health, Inc., New York).

Levinson, H. "What Work Means to A Man," *Think,* January-February 1964, p. 7.

Luton, F. H. "An Alumni Club Carries On Where the Hospital Left Off," *Mental Hospitals.* August 1961, Vol. 12, p. 24. *The Journal of Hospital and Community Psychiatry* (American Psychiatric Association, Washington, D.C.).

Olshansky, S. "Passing: Road to Normalization for Ex Mental Patients," *Mental Hygiene.* January 1966, Vol. 50, No. 1, p. 86. (National Association for Mental Health, Inc., New York).

Ozarin, L. D. "The Community Mental Health Center: A Public Health Facility," *American Journal of Public Health.* January 1966, Vol. 56, No. 1.

Patterson, C. H. "A Suggested Blueprint for Psychiatric Rehabilitation," *Community Mental Health Journal.* Spring 1965, Vol. I, No. 1.

Titmuss, R. M. "Community Care of the Mentally Ill: Some British Observations," *Canada's Mental Health.* November-December 1965, Supplement No. 49 (Department of National Health and Welfare, Ottawa, Canada).

United States Department of Health, Education, and Welfare, Vocational Rehabilitation Administration. "Helping the Mentally Ill: Rehabilitation Program in a State Hospital: Doorway to life—A Halfway House; The Mental Patient Who *Wants* to Fail; Workshop for Chronic Mental Patients; Hospitalizing the Mentally Ill," selected articles from back issues of *The Rehabilitation Record* (Washington, D.C.), July-August 1961.

Whatley, C. D., Jr. "Employer Attitudes: Discharged Patients and Job Durability," *Mental Hygiene,* January 1964, Vol. 48, No. 1, p. 121. (National Association for Mental Health, Inc. New York).

Zolik, E. S., Lantz, E. M. "A Comparative Study of Return Rates to Two Mental Hospitals," *Community Mental Health Journal.* Fall 1965, Vol. II, No. 3, p. 233. (Boston, Mass.).

REPORTS

American Medical Association, Council on Occupational Health. "Guide for Evaluating Employability After Psychiatric Illness," (reprint), *Journal of American Medical Association.* September 22, 1962, Vol. 181.

American Psychiatric Association. "From the Ward Into the World," Miller, D., Barnhouse, R. *Psychiatric Studies and Projects.* December 1965, Vol. 3, No. 8.

American Psychiatric Association. "Post-Hospital Evaluation of Psychiatric Patients: The Social Adjustment Inventory Method," December 1964, Vol. II, No. 15, *Psychiatric Studies and Projects* (Washington, D.C.).

American Psychological Association. "Social Therapy, Resocialization and Psychiatric Adjustment: A Symposium Presented at the Convention of the American Psychological Association, August 30, 1963, Philadelphia, Pa.," Washington, D.C.

Commonwealth of Pennsylvania, 1965-1966 Budget, General Fund, Submitted to the General Assembly by William W. Scranton, Governor, February 7, 1966, Harrisburg, Pa.

Commonwealth of Pennsylvania. "The Comprehensive Mental Health Plan," C. J. Bodarky, Ed. (Health and Welfare Building, Harrisburg, Pa.) 1965.

Commonwealth of Pennsylvania, Department of Internal Affairs. *Pennsylvania Statistical Abstract: 1964-65,* 7th Annual Edition (Harrisburg, Pa.).

Commonwealth of Pennsylvania, Department of Public Welfare, Office of Mental Health. Position paper: "Rehabilitation and Aftercare for Mentally Ill and Emotionally Disturbed Adults," October 1964 (Harrisburg, Pa.) p. 1.

Commonwealth of Pennsylvania, Department of Public Welfare, Office of Mental Health. "Regional Committee Reports" (Harrisburg, Pa.).

Hogg Foundation for Mental Health, University of Texas. "After Hospitalization: The Mental Patient and His Family," Simmons, O. G. (Austin, Texas), 1960.

Joint Information Service, American Psychiatric Association, and The National Association for Mental Health, Inc. "The Community Mental Health Center: An Analysis of Existing Models," Glasscote, R., Sanders, D., Forstenzer, H. M., Foley, A. R. (Washington, D.C.) September 1964.

Joint Information Service, American Psychiatric Association, and The National Association for Mental Health, Inc. "Fifteen Indices: An Aid in Reviewing State and Local Mental Health and Hospital Programs," (Washington, D.C.) February 1964.

Louisiana Association for Mental Health. "The Social Club: A Bridge from Mental Hospital to Community," Palmer, M. (New Orleans, La.).

Mental Health Association of Erie County, Aftercare Committee. "A Program to Provide Psychotropic Medications to the Impoverished Mentally Ill." (Erie, Pa.) October 1965.

Mental Health Association of St. Louis. "A Rehabilitation Facility in Transition: A Case History of the St. Louis Halfway House." (St. Louis, Mo.) December 1965.

The National Association for Mental Health, Inc. "Report of the Consultation on Rehabilitation and Aftercare, Sponsored by

155

The National Association for Mental Health, Inc." New York, May 14-15, 1962.

National Institute of Mental Health. "Community Mental Health Advances," U.S. Department of Health, Education and Welfare, Public Health Service (Washington, D.C.) April 1964, pp. 1-8.

National Institute of Mental Health. "Patients in Mental Institutions, 1963. Part II," U. S. Department of Health, Education, and Welfare, Public Health Service, Biometrics Branch (Washington, D.C.).

National Institute of Mental Health. "Provisional Patient Movement and Administrative Data, State and County Mental Hospitals, United States." (Bethesda, Md.) January 1964.

National Institute of Mental Health. "Patients in Mental Institutions, 1962, Part II. State and County Mental Hospitals," (Washington: U.S. Government Printing Office) 1964, pp. II-8, II-9.

National Institute of Mental Health. "Research Activities." (Bethesda, Md.) December 1964, p. 7.

New York State Department of Mental Hygiene, Mental Health Research Unit. "Study of Community Mental Health Clinics. Report I: Characteristics of Patients Applying for Service, and Factors Determining Acceptance for Treatment," Cumming, J., Saenger, G. (Syracuse, N.Y.) October 1965.

Pennsylvania Mental Health, Inc. "A Profile of the Eighteen State Mental Hospitals in Pennsylvania." (Philadelphia, Pa.) February 1965.

Pennsylvania Mental Health, Inc. "What Every Mental Health Association Director Should Know About the Regional Committee Reports of the Comprehensive Mental Health Plan. (Philadelphia, Pa.) September 1965.

Pennsylvania Mental Health, Inc. "What Every Mental Health Association Director Should Know About The Task Force Reports: Implications for Local Program and Action." (Philadelphia, Pa.) April 28, 1965.

Southern Regional Education Board. "Professionals' Views on the Need for Psychiatric Aftercare Services; Aftercare: Report of a Conference on an Assessment of Needs and Problems in Aftercare," G. H. Wolkon, and H. Tanaka, Eds. Penningroth, P. W., Sparer, D. *Mental Health Rehabilitation Research, Technical Report Series VI,* (Atlanta, Ga.) October 1963.

State of California, Department of Mental Hygiene. "Annual Report." (Sacramento, Calif.) 1944.

State of California, Department of Mental Hygiene, Bureau of Research. "Worlds that Fail: Part I. Retrospective Analysis of Mental Patients' Careers," Miller, D. *California Mental Health Research Monograph No. 6,* (Sacramento, Calif.) 1965.

State of California, Department of Mental Hygiene. Bureau of Research, "Worlds That Fail: Part II. Disbanded Worlds: A Study of Returns to the Mental Hospital," Miller, D., Dawson, W. *California Mental Health Research Monograph No. 7,* (Sacramento, Calif.) 1965.

United Mental Health Services of Allegheny County, Inc. "A Study of Patterns of Service to Persons Following Psychiatric Hospitalization in Allegheny County, Pennsylvania," Strecker, M. C., Dean, C. W., (Pittsburgh, Pa.) April 1964.

United States Congress, House Subcommittee of the Committee on Interstate and Foreign Commerce, *Hearings,* H. R., 3688, 88th Congress, First Session, March 26, 27 and 28, 1963, p. 78.

United States Department of Health, Education, and Welfare. "Mental Health Activities and the Development of Comprehensive Health Programs in the Community: Report of the Surgeon General's Ad Hoc Committee on Mental Health Activities," August 1962.

PAMPHLETS AND MONOGRAPHS

"Community Mental Health Advances," U.S. Department of Health, Education, and Welfare, Public Health Service, National Institute of Mental Health (Bethesda, Md.) April 1964.

"The Community Mental Health Centers Act (1963): A Commentary," U.S. Department of Health, Education, and Welfare, Public Health Service, National Institute of Mental Health (Bethesda, Md.) No. 1298.

"Comprehensive Psychiatric Programs: A Survey of 234 Facilities," Joint Information Service, American Psychiatric Association, and The National Association for Mental Health, Inc. (Washington, D.C.) June 1963.

"Concept and Challenge: The Comprehensive Community Mental Health Center," U.S. Department of Health, Education, and Welfare, Public Health Service, National Institute of Mental Health (Bethesda, Md.) April 1964.

Halpert, H. P. "Public Opinions and Attitudes About Mental Health," Research Utilization Series, U.S. Department of Health, Education, and Welfare, May 1963.

Harrison, E. "Mental Aftercare: Assignment for the Sixties," *Public Affairs Pamphlet,* No. 318 (New York), Public Affairs Pamphlet, 1961.

Jacob, N. P. "Why Do Community Psychiatric Clinics Reject Patients?" Paper presented at Annual Meeting, American Orthopsychiatric Association, New York, N.Y., March 19, 1965.

"Lifeline: Aftercare," Smith Kline and French Laboratories (1500 Spring Garden St., Philadelphia, Pa. 19101) 1962.

"Mental Health Education: A Critique," Pennsylvania Mental Health, Inc. (Philadelphia, Pa.) May 1960.

"Network: A Report on Coordinating Psychiatric Aftercare Services," Pennsylvania Mental Health, Inc. (Philadelphia, Pa.) April 1957.

"Rehabilitating the Mentally Ill," U.S. Department of Health, Education, and Welfare, Vocational Rehabilitation Administration (Washington, D.C.) October 1964.

Thompson, D. B. "Guide to Job Placement of the Mentally Restored," President's Committee on Employment of the Handicapped (Washington, D.C.) 1965.

Wilson, R. N. "Coming Home: The Problem of Aftercare," Southern Regional Education Board (Atlanta, Ga.) 1965.

Date Due